The Complete Guide to Make-up

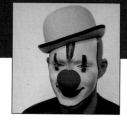
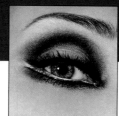
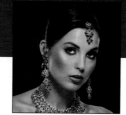
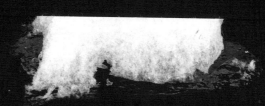

HAIRDRESSING AND BEAUTY INDUSTRY AUTHORITY SERIES

HAIRDRESSING

Mahogany Hairdressing: Steps to Cutting, Colouring and Finishing Hair *Martin Gannon and Richard Thompson*

Mahogany Hairdressing: Advanced Looks *Richard Thompson and Martin Gannon*

Essensuals, Next Generation Toni & Guy: Step by Step

Professional Men's Hairdressing *Guy Kremer and Jacki Wadeson*

The Art of Dressing Long Hair *Guy Kremer and Jacki Wadeson*

Patrick Cameron: Dressing Long Hair *Patrick Cameron and Jacki Wadeson*

Patrick Cameron: Dressing Long Hair Book 2 *Patrick Cameron*

Bridal Hair *Pat Dixon and Jacki Wadeson*

Trevor Sorbie: The Bridal Hair Book *Trevor Sorbie and Jacki Wadeson*

Trevor Sorbie: Visions in Hair *Kris Sorbie and Jacki Wadeson*

The Total Look: The Style Guide for Hair and Make-Up Professionals *Ian Mistlin*

Art of Hair Colouring *David Adams and Jacki Wadeson*

Begin Hairdressing: The Official Guide to Level 1 *Martin Green*

Hairdressing – The Foundations: The official Guide to S/NVQ Level 2 5e *Leo Palladino and Martin Green*

Professional Hairdressing: The Official Guide to Level 3 4e *Martin Green and Leo Palladino*

Men's Hairdressing: Traditional and Modern Barbering 2e *Maurice Lister*

African-Caribbean Hairdressing 2e *Sandra Gittens*

Salon Management *Martin Green*

eXtensions: The Official Guide to Hair Extensions *Theresa Bullock*

The Colour Book: The Official Guide to Colour at NVQ Levels 2 & 3 *Tracey Lloyd with Christine McMillan-Bodell*

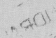

BEAUTY THERAPY

Beauty Basics – The Official Guide to Level 1 *Lorraine Nordmann*

Beauty Therapy – The Foundations: The Official Guide to Level 2 *Lorraine Nordmann*

Professional Beauty Therapy: The Official Guide to Level 3 *Lorraine Nordmann, Lorraine Williamson, Pamela Linforth and Jo Crowder*

Aromatherapy for the Beauty Therapist *Valerie Ann Worwood*

Indian Head Massage *Muriel Burnham-Airey and Adele O'Keefe*

The Official Guide to Body Massage *Adele O'Keefe*

An Holistic Guide to Anatomy and Physiology *Tina Parsons*

The Encyclopedia of Nails *Jacqui Jefford and Anne Swain*

Nail Artistry *Jacqui Jefford, Sue Marsh and Anne Swain*

The Complete Nail Technician *Marian Newman*

The World of Skin Care: A Scientific Companion *Dr John Gray*

An Holistic Guide to Reflexology *Tina Parsons*

Nutrition: A Practical Approach *Suzanne Le Quesne*

An Holistic Guide to Massage *Tina Parsons*

The Spa Book: The Official Guide to Spa Therapy *Jane Crebbin-Bailey, Dr John Harcup and John Harrington*

The Complete Guide to Make-up *Suzanne Le Quesne*

The Complete Make-up Artist: Working in Film, Fashion, Television and Theatre *Penny Delamar*

The Essential Guide to Holistic & Complementary Therapy *Helen Beckmann and Suzanne Le Quesne*

The Complete Guide to Make-up

The Official Guide to Make-up at Levels 2 and 3

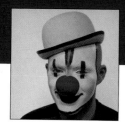
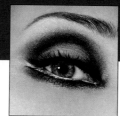
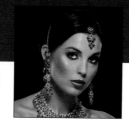

SUZANNE LE QUESNE

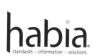

DELMAR
CENGAGE Learning™

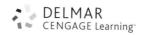

Australia • Brazil • Japan • Korea • Mexico • Singapore • Spain • United Kingdom • United States

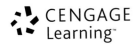

The Complete Guide to Make-up: The Official Guide to Make-Up at Levels 2 and 3
Suzanne Le Quesne

Publisher: Lucy Mills

Production Editor: Alissa Chappell

Editorial Assistant: Rebecca Hussey

Head of Manufacturing: Jane Glendening

Production Controller: Tom Relf

Marketing Manager: Jason Bennett

Typesetter: Meridian Colour Repro Ltd

Cover design: Jackie Wrout

Text design: Design Deluxe, Bath, UK

For product information and technology assistance, contact **emea.info@cengage.com**.

For permission to use material from this text or product, and for permission queries, email **clsuk.permissions@cengage.com**.

The Author has asserted the right under the Copyright, Designs and Patents Act 1988 to be identified as Author of this Work.

British Library Cataloguing-in-Publication Data
A catalogue record for this book is available from the British Library.

ISBN: 978-1-84480-144-2

Cengage Learning EMEA
Cheriton House, North Way, Andover, Hampshire, SP10 5BE, United Kingdom

Cengage Learning products are represented in Canada by Nelson Education Ltd.

For your lifelong learning solutions, visit **www.cengage.co.uk**

Purchase your next print book, e-book or e-chapter at **www.ichapters.co.uk**

Printed by Seng Lee Press, Singapore
5 6 7 8 9 10 – 11 10 09

contents

acknowledgements

It was an honour to be asked to write this book for Cengage Learning, but I knew that the only way I was going to complete it to their high standards, was to call in lots of favours and to ask for lots of help! Accordingly, I am indebted to many people for their help, guidance and patience during the writing of this book. First to the book's sponsors: Stephen Clennel, Managing Director of Anthony Braden Cosmetics, Tim Rice, Managing Director of Black by Design Make-Up and Mike, Anne and Carl King from The Three Kings Make-Up Supplies. My sponsors supported me throughout the writing of the book and gave me so much of their valuable knowledge, expertise and time that I am truly indebted to them. I would like to thank all the make-up artists, the face and body painters and the airbrush and henna artists who all worked so hard in compiling the looks, many of whom began as work colleagues and ended up as good friends.

There are always, of course, certain people to whom no amount of acknowledgement or thanks would ever be enough. These are the people who live with authors – the partners and family members who have to live with the highs and lows of someone writing a book. My very special thanks goes to my fantastic husband Barry, who was always there looking after me and listening to my endless ramblings about 'the Book'.

There are special friends too, without whose help this book would never have been completed. Tamsin Pyne, fellow make-up artist and good friend, not only completed some great make-up looks for the book, but also spent hours proofreading and editing the text, and undertaking such a momentous task with great humour! I will forever be indebted to her. I will never forget the enthusiasm of Shabana Begum, the make-up artist for Mendhi/Henna, who not only gave hours of her time helping me but brought fun and laughter to the photo shoots. Alison Wolstenholme, airbrush artist, was of immense help also. Other make-up artists and friends who have given me much support are Adele Palmer, Dorinda Sweales, Ema Louise Doherty, Pippa Haye, Ann Eatwell, Paula Southern, Sue Callaghan and Judie Becque. Special thanks must go to Donna Jones for her participation in the camouflage chapter, and Emma Louise Watson (Jersey), for my new PR photo! I would also like to sincerely thank Andy Donley, fellow National Make-up Competition Judge, for his contribution to the research and worksheets chapter and for his excellent contribution of the Halloween make-up.

Thanks are also due to our photographers. Barry Le Quesne took most of the theatrical pictures with a digital camera. But credit must be given to our main photographer Myk from The Bakery Photographic Studios, who besides taking some great shots for the fashion and photographic sections of the book, and the majority of the product shots, taught me patience! Just as you can't hurry a good make-up, Myk taught us that you can't hurry a good photograph either. Thank you too to Vanessa Wayne, not only for her make-up skills, but also for her photographic skills.

Thanks also go to DSH Hire, Farnborough, (+44) 01252 518777 (www.dshhire.co.uk) for the loan of the stage lighting and rostrum.

Lastly, a big thank you to all the models who so patiently sat through, sometimes very long, make-up sessions – without you this book could not have been completed.

Thanks again to everyone.

about the author

With eighteen years experience in the health and beauty business, Suzanne Le Quesne has become a leading authority on beauty and holistic therapies. The Le Quesne Academy, Suzanne's training school (established in 1987) is a highly respected training centre for holistic and beauty therapies with the Fashion and Photographic Make-Up Diploma being the school's flagship course.

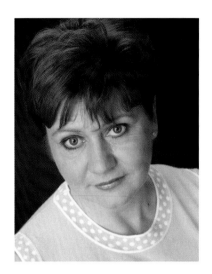

Suzanne's first serious encounter with make-up was in 1985 when she attended the Joan Price Face Place in London for an intensive course covering all types of make-up application and photographic work. That was enough to get her hooked and she has been involved in make-up ever since. From teaching in colleges, working with photographers for portrait work, organising major charity make-up/fashion events, to planning and executing the Fashion and Photographic Make-Up Diploma she now teaches in the UK and Spain. From 1987 to 1997 Suzanne was a practising therapist in her own salon in the Channel Islands. Her flourishing career meant a move to the UK in 2001 where she worked with her husband in their private holistic clinic in Shropshire. Having written five books in four years, Suzanne's time is now free to return to running her training schools in the UK and Spain, where she now lives with her husband, Barry.

Suzanne is frequently asked to judge major national make-up competitions on behalf of *Professional Beauty* magazine and The Association of Therapy Lecturers. She is a leading authority on nutrition and is an established author, speaker and broadcaster.

By the same author:

Nutrition – A Practical Approach for Holistic Therapists
Health & Beauty Enterprises – 2001, reprinted 2002

Nutrition – A Practical Approach
Cengage Learning – 2003, reprinted 2004

The pH Diet
(with Bharti Vyas) Thorsons – 2004

The Complete Guide to Complementary Therapy
Cengage Learning – 2004

introduction

The desire to wear make-up is not new; on the contrary, there is evidence throughout history of ancient peoples adorning themselves with colour. Different cultures developed many ways of applying make-up on the face and body for a variety of reasons; to enhance beauty, to cover defects, or to take on parts of characters in the theatrical plays of their times. Colour was always important. The Egyptians used black kohl, vegetable dyes, red clay and toxic white lead, which were all used to adorn the faces of both sexes, whereas medieval women used white lead to achieve the complexion that was the fashion of the day. Now, in the twenty-first century, with safer products for everyone, huge colour ranges for fashion and, with new innovative materials, fantastic special effects and camouflage products available for film and television make-overs, the world of make-up and colour is as exciting as ever.

The aims of this book are twofold. I will guide you through the many and varied practical skills required to be competent in all areas of make-up application, from general straight make-up for beauty salons and retail outlets, to make-up suitable for film, fashion, pop videos, television and theatre.

Secondly, I will advise you on effective ways of searching for and obtaining work in your chosen specialised area of make-up. Many students leave college not knowing clearly what to do to start off their career. This can result in them making fundamental errors and working for years receiving little or no money. However, there *are* times when working for nothing has advantages. Working with photographers and models whilst putting together your professional portfolio, your 'Book', is one example of working without payment. However, as it is *only* on the strength of your 'Book' that you will find employment, this type of unpaid work is more than acceptable. I will give you valuable advice about which photographs to include and which to omit from your 'Book' to make the most impact, and in what order to write your CV when applying for work.

Being a make-up artist is not an easy option; it requires hard work, enthusiasm and patience. A make-up artist's job not only involves putting make-up on other people in order to change their appearance, but also includes general beauty therapy and hairdressing techniques. Techniques such as eyelash tinting and perming, eyebrow shaping, facial cleansing, toning and moisturising, enhancing a model's nails and hair, general hairdressing and cleaning and styling wigs can all be expected of a make-up artist. The more of these skills you have, the more work will be available to you.

Being a make-up artist usually involves making up actors, actresses, models or presenters for television, video, film, theatre or fashion. This may involve making the person look their best in front of the cameras or audience by simply using stronger or more suitable colours for the occasion, applying powder to hide shine or merely styling hair. Make-up is such a diverse topic that after basic training (NVQ Level 2), many students go on to specialise in one particular area. Specialisms include theatrical and media make-up, fashion and photographic make-up, and camouflage make-up (NVQ Level 3).

Theatrical and media make-up may involve creating special effects such as ageing, scars or wounds, or recreating historical looks for period productions. You may also be required to apply facial hair and/or prosthetics to achieve the full effect of a particular look. A fashion make-up artist, on the other hand, tends to specialise in magazine work, fashion, catwalk shows and pop promotions. Career goals may be to make-up the model for a front cover of a prestigious magazine or be on a make-up team for the London, Milan or New York Fashion Weeks, or even the latest pop video. A camouflage make-up artist may work in more of a medical environment.

Whichever area of make-up you want to work in, the one qualification you will need, more than any other, is the key skill of communication. All make-up artists work closely with other professionals – photographers, hair stylists, editors, directors, visual effects supervisors, agents and models – and your ability to communicate well is fundamental.

foreword

With new standards, more public interest, and a growing share of the beauty market, there has never been a better time to get involved in make-up.

And with that, there is a need for a book that covers the entire scope of make-up to help those just starting out, whether they are students beginning their career or working beauty therapists looking to extend their services and range of skills.

Who better to write that book than Suzanne Le Quesne?

Suzanne is one of the UK's leading authorities on make-up, having worked in the industry for nearly 20 years, established her own training academy and judged make-up competitions throughout the world.

Having authored five books in four years, Suzanne is a proven communicator with a track record in producing educational texts that are interesting, involving and informative.

I have no doubt that, like her other books, The Complete Guide to Make-Up will prove to be an invaluable resource to learner and educator alike.

Alan Goldsbro
CEO HABIA

chapter 1

Understanding colour

An exciting part of our work is to be aware of each new season's colours and products, designers and fashions, models and photographers, special effects films and new theatrical productions. However, to really appreciate these, you need a thorough understanding of colour, application, technique and other connected aspects of your trade. These aspects, at first glance, may not appear exciting in themselves, but they are nevertheless fundamental to your career. Understanding colour, the first of these basic requirements in studying make-up, is covered in this chapter. The study of colour can be complex and sometimes confusing but, as you work through the exercises, you will come to appreciate its importance and relationship to your work as a make-up artist.

Learning objectives

In this chapter you will learn about:

- **light and colour**
- **coloured light and coloured pigment**
- **the classification and characteristics of pigment colours**
- **primary, secondary and tertiary colours**
- **complementary colours**
- **warm and cool colours**
- **the psychological effects of colour**
- **hue, brightness, tone and saturation**
- **tints and shades**
- **harmony and contrast**
- **skin tones**
- **how to make corrections to skin colour**
- **lighting for film and photography**

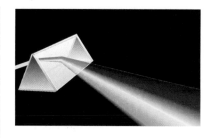

Light being passed through a
glass prism

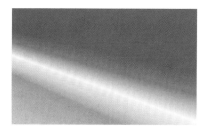

The colour spectrum

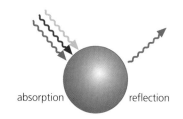

absorption   reflection

Absorption of light

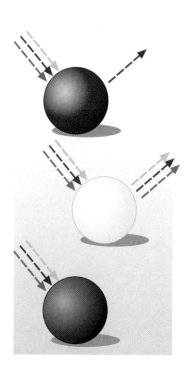

How light is absorbed or
reflected by surfaces

LIGHT

The theories concerning the nature of light reveal that it is a form of
electromagnetic energy and that it travels in the form of waves. The eye is
able to perceive colour because each colour has a different wavelength. Red
colours have the longest wavelengths and blue colours the shortest. When
light is passed through a glass prism, its waves split according to their length
and can be 'seen' as separate colours – red, orange, yellow, green, blue,
indigo and violet – always in that order. This can be remembered by using
the acronym: ROY G BIV. A natural example is a rainbow. Collectively these
colours are known as the **colour spectrum**. All other colours are variations
of these seven basic colours.

Vision is stimulated by light; it allows us to see the characteristics of objects.
Light is absorbed or reflected by the surface of the object. The colour we see
depends on how much light is reflected and how much is absorbed. The
reflected light shows the object's colour. If most of the light is reflected we see
'white' and if most is absorbed we see 'black'. So something looks the colour
it does because it reflects the colour we see and absorbs all the other colours.

Light is a crucial factor for a make-up professional. It is important to study
light (natural, artificial, soft or intense) when identifying skin type, colour
and tone and also when choosing the texture of products to be used from
light tinted moisturisers – soft products – to pan sticks – hard products.
Natural light makes colours more noticeable. For this reason, with natural
light you can use soft, warm colours, and soft and light textured products.
Conversely with artificial light you may use more intense colours and a more
heavily textured product.

COLOUR

In everyday life, colour acts as a source of information helping us to
distinguish things. Just think of the chaos if traffic lights were colourless! In
make-up, a knowledge of colour and the application of its theories help us to:

- *select* the correct make-up to conceal, highlight, shade and colour to
  achieve the intended result;
- *intensify* the colour of lips and eyes;
- *illuminate* the face;
- *correct* imperfections on the skin;
- *identify* natural skin colours, tones and undertones.

LIGHT COLOUR AND PIGMENT COLOUR

Most people are aware that primary colours can be mixed to produce all
other colours. However, not everyone is aware that primary colours can be
split into two categories – additive and subtractive.

'Light colour' is the colour that comes from *natural sources* such as the sun, *or* from *artificial sources* of light such as a light bulb. Mixed natural light colours create brightness, this phenomenon is called the *additive* mixture. Red, green and blue colours of natural light are called pure colours and are the additive primaries. If you mix them equally you will get white.

A pigment is a substance which gives colour to the objects it is applied to and which can absorb or reflect lengths of waves. In comparison to light colours, the pigment colours *subtract* each other's **chromatic** qualities when mixed. The end result of a mixture of *pigment* colours is called a *subtractive* mixture. The subtractive primaries are red, blue and yellow. These are used when mixing pigments.

Red, yellow and blue are, therefore, commonly known as the primary pigment colours. If you mix them equally you will get a very dark grey, or black.

As make-up involves pigment colours, these subtractive mixtures are important and you need to be familiar with the variety of colours which can be made from the three primaries.

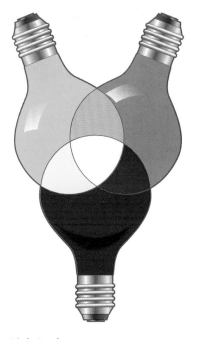

'Light' colour

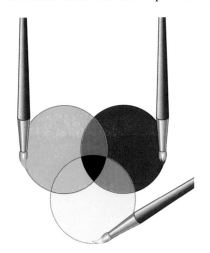

'Pigment' colour

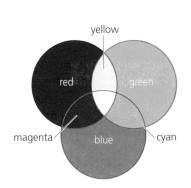

The primary colours of light

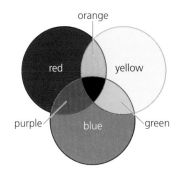

The primary colours of pigment

CLASSIFICATION AND CHARACTERISTICS OF PIGMENT COLOURS

Primary colours

Primary colours are pure colours, with no mixture of any other colour.

The *pigment* primary colours are red (magenta), yellow (cadmium) and blue (cyan).

Secondary colours

Secondary colours are produced when you mix two primary colours. The secondary colours created by equal amounts of two primary colours are orange, green and violet. These secondary colours are said to be midway between the primary colours.

Obtaining secondary colours

Two primary colours mixed together	The resulting secondary colour
Red + Yellow	Orange
Yellow + Blue	Green
Blue + Red	Violet

An important point to note is that you cannot mix any shade of colour. It is therefore quite difficult to make white light or black pigment by mixing the relative primaries because you have to have the *exact* primary colours of light or paint in order for this to work. You therefore need to start with 'true' primary colours (primary colours not mixed with any other colour). Making a bright green with yellow and a royal blue is impossible as the royal blue also contains some red, so you will be trying to make a secondary green with three colours.

STUDENT ACTIVITY

1.1 Making secondary colours from primary colours

Have a look at the example on the left and complete the circle on the right. Use colours as close to true primary colours as you can – cyan blue, magenta red and cadmium yellow. Paradise Aqua colours in dark blue, red and yellow, are excellent for this exercise.

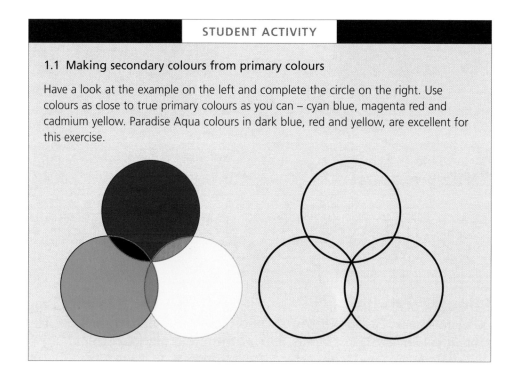

1.2 The colour wheel

1 Draw a circle and divide it into six equal sections – as in the illustration.

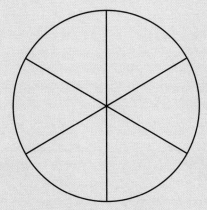

2 Paint (or colour) each alternative section with each of the primary colours – red, blue and yellow.

3 Mix a little blue with red. Fill in the section between the red and the blue with the colour you made – it will be violet, the particular violet you will get will depend on how much red and how much blue you used.

4 Now try mixing blue and yellow. Colour the section between the blue and the yellow with the colour you made, which will be green. Again, the particular green will depend on how much blue and yellow you used.

5 Finally mix red and yellow and you will get orange. Colour the final section of your colour wheel with the orange, the depth of which will again depend on the quantities of red and yellow you used.

Tertiary colours

Tertiary colours are made from a mixture of one primary colour and one secondary colour.

Obtaining tertiary colours

One primary colour + one of its secondary colours mixed together	The resulting tertiary colour
Primary Blue + Secondary Green	Blue-green
Primary Yellow + Secondary Green	Olive (yellowish-green)
Primary Blue + Secondary Violet	Purplish-blue
Primary Red + Secondary Violet	Carmine (dark red)
Primary Red + Secondary Orange	Vermilion (bright red)

Tertiary colours can also be made by mixing all three primary colours together, which creates colours that tend to be earthy tones. Browns and khakis are examples of tertiary colours mixed together with *different proportions* of primary colours.

COMPLEMENTARY COLOURS

Complementary colours are those which are opposite each other on the colour wheel. For example, red is opposite (complementary to) green. Green is made from the *other* two primary colours, so it contains no red.

1.3 Complete the sequences below.

1 The first sequence represents making secondary colours, the first has been done for you.

2 The second sequence represents primary colours and secondary colours. Using paint or colour, mix the colours and complete the sequences (reserve portions of violet, green and orange).

3 The third sequence represents primary colours and secondary colours, again complete the sequences. What will you call each of the tertiary colours? Invent names for them (olive green, warm yellow, etc.).

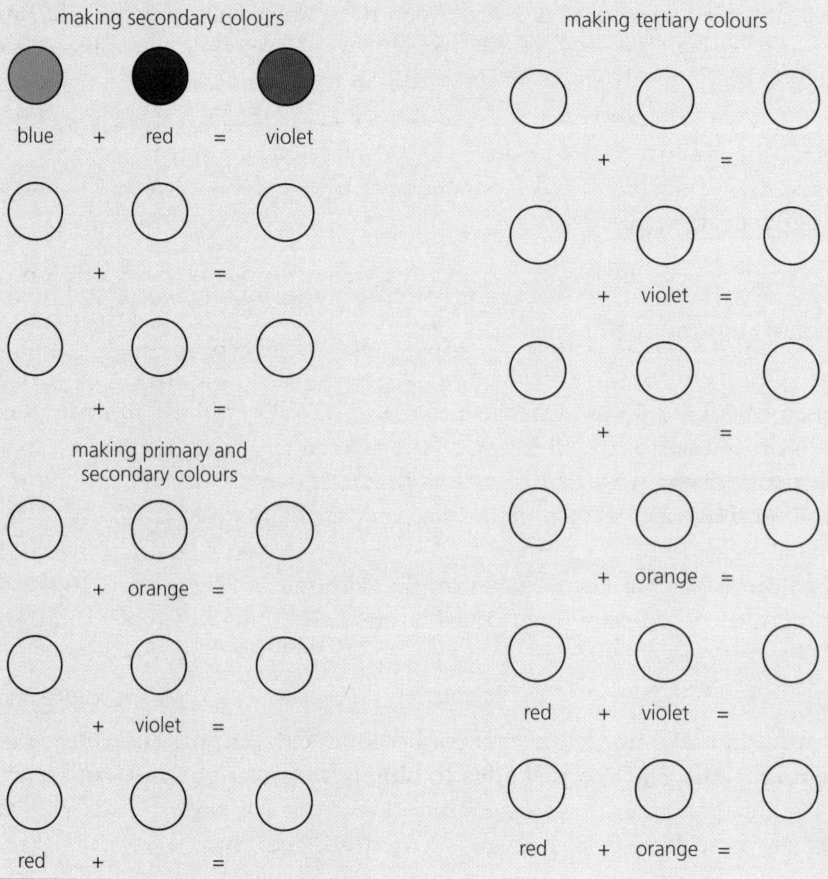

making secondary colours

blue   +   red   =   violet

+   =

+   =

making primary and
secondary colours

+   orange   =

+   violet   =

red   +   =

making tertiary colours

+   =

+   violet   =

+   =

+   orange   =

red   +   violet   =

red   +   orange   =

Therefore the primary colour that does *not* take part in the mixture is the complementary colour of the secondary colour. For example: violet is the complementary of yellow, because it is obtained by mixing blue and red. It is because the primary colour yellow is *not* in the original mix that violet becomes its complementary colour.

Therefore:

- orange (red and yellow) is the complementary of blue
- green (yellow and blue) is the complementary of red
- violet (red and blue) is the complementary of yellow

Each primary has a secondary colour which is its complementary and vice versa.

Tertiary colours also have complementary colours, but in these cases the opposite colour is also a tertiary colour:

- yellow-orange is the complementary of blue-violet
- yellow-green is the complementary of red-violet
- red-orange is the complementary of blue-green, etc.

WARM AND COOL COLOURS

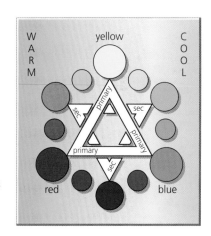

The colour wheel

You may have heard of warm and cool colours in connection with clothes, home decorating and other aspects of colour. If we draw a line through the chromatic circle of colours, it can be seen that the colours can be split into two groups: red-yellow colours (where warmth dominates) and blue colours (where coolness dominates). The colours on the right of the wheel shown here are known as cool colours – colours which are blue or have a leaning towards blue (yellow-green to blue-violet). The colours on the left are known as warm colours – colours which are red or have a leaning towards red (yellow-orange to red-violet).

This concept is very important in any area where colour is used, but it is especially so in make-up application where the correct choice and use of warm and cool colours is vital. If colours are unflattering to a face it may be because you have chosen the wrong colours. For example, you may have chosen cool colours when warm ones would have been more appropriate for the skin colour/tone/undertone of the model, or vice versa, or you may have used both warm and cool colours that may not create a harmonious result. Therefore, it is always recommended, at the beginning of your training at least, to be committed to completing a make-up in either cool *or* warm colours, but *not* both. For example, with natural light, warm tones are recommended, whereas with artificial light or at night, cool tones can be used. Once you have experience and understand the concept of warm and cool colours, then you can experiment!

When used in make-up, warm and cool colours can emphasise features, for instance they can give warm shades to blue eyes and cool shades to brown eyes. They can also help to create a mood – if warm tones are used with the correct props and lighting, a warm, sunny, Caribbean beach scene can be created even on a cloudy day in the UK!

THE PSYCHOLOGICAL EFFECTS OF COLOUR

Different studies have demonstrated that colours have a great influence on a person's psychology. This means that colours can affect people's minds positively or negatively, depending on how they are used. While some colours, like red, are stimulants, other colours, like blue, are calming.

- stimulant colours – warm colours, result in excitement.
- sedative colours – cool colours, generate a sense of calm and tranquillity.

HUE, BRIGHTNESS, TONE AND SATURATION

Hue

The term **hue** is used when describing a colour and represents the differences between colours – red, blue, yellow and so forth are all 'hues' of colour. Grey cannot be described as a 'hue' because it is a mixture of black and white – both of which are not in the colour spectrum. Therefore, only colours originating from the colour spectrum can be described as having a hue.

Brightness

Brightness represents the range from light to dark. The pure primary colours are the brightest. The brightness scale runs from any light variation of a colour to its dark variation. The scale of greys is simple because there are no hues. The darkness or lightness of a colour – its position on the scale – is called its value. A light colour has a high value while a dark colour has a low value.

Tone

According to its **tone**, a colour can be classified as light, medium or dark.

Saturation

Saturation is the level of purity of a colour. A colour is never pure if mixed with white. Therefore, the more white there is in a colour, the less saturated it is. For instance, pink and sky blue are *low saturation* colours because there is more white in the colour than the red or blue they originated from. Conversely, pure red, green or blue colours are saturated.

TINTS AND SHADES

We now have twelve colours on our colour wheel (including all the primary, secondary and tertiary colours). Each of these individual colours is a hue, because they contain no black or white. You can change the saturation of a hue by adding white (lightness) or black (shadow). The amount of saturation gives us tints and shades. For example, pink will be a **tint** because it is the result of adding white to red. In the same way you can add white to any colour and the colour will get lighter.

If you wanted to make any hue darker, you would add black, resulting in a darker colour or a **shade**.

STUDENT ACTIVITY

1.4   Saturation and brightness

A practice exercise for two of the most important features or qualities of colour – saturation and brightness. If you mix a colour with white, you will see that the colour saturation diminishes. When you mix a colour with black it becomes darker – less bright. Using true colours (primary colours not mixed with any other colour) mix each in proportion as indicated to discover the effects for yourself.

100% black	75% black + 25% cyan	50% black + 50% cyan	25% black + 75% cyan	100% cyan	25% white + 75%cyan	50% white + 50%cyan	75% white + 25%cyan	100% white

100% black	75% black + 25%yellow	50% black + 50%yellow	25% black + 75%yellow	100% yellow	25% white + 75%yellow	50% white + 50%yellow	75% white + 25%yellow	100% white

100% black	75% black + 25% red	50% black + 50% red	25% black + 75% red	100% red	25% white + 75% red	50% white + 50% red	75% white + 25% red	100% white

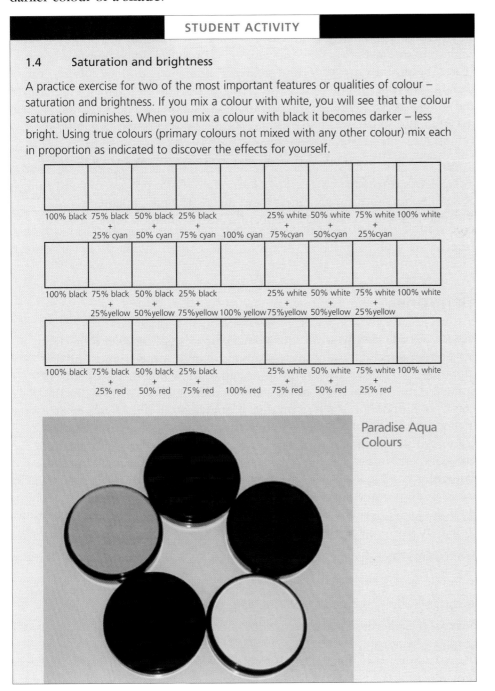

Paradise Aqua
Colours

THE APPLICATIONS OF COLOUR IN MAKE-UP

Harmony and contrast

There are no hard and fast rules with reference to make-up application. This is because styles and preferences may change according to fashion. Therefore, colour combinations that are considered to be 'horrible' at the moment could become fashionable next season. Despite that, a professional in make-up must be aware of the principles of harmony and contrast even though we may sometimes deliberately break the rules!

Harmony occurs when all the chosen colours 'go well together' and can be achieved using similar or contrasting colours. In make-up you should try to achieve harmony between all the products you select, for example eye shadows, blushers, bronzers and shaders, highlighters and lip colours. You should also take into consideration elements such as the shape of the face, the colour of eyes, complexion, the model's personality, the occasion for the make-up and so on. Harmony should also be understood as something changeable – like fashion and time.

Contrast is achieved by bringing together colours that are *opposite* to each other in the chromatic circle (the colour wheel). The process of contrasting allows certain interesting elements and details to be highlighted. Asymmetries and certain negative features can be hidden through contrasting.

Skin tones

Before you can start to work on any make-up design, the skin tone (light, medium or dark) and undertones (yellow, orange and red) must first be identified. No matter how well you design it, the whole make-up may be spoiled if the identification of skin tone and undertone is wrong, as the choice of foundation is based on this. Identifying the right tones of the skin is therefore crucial to obtaining the desired look. There are three basic colours of skin: white, brown and black, three basic tones: light, medium and dark, and three basic undertones: yellow, orange and red – but there are numerous combinations. Observation is the best method of ascertaining skin tone, and this will come with experience. All skins, like all people, are different and it is very common to have to mix various colours of foundation to get the exact match you need.

White skins often have:

- visible signs of redness
- thinner skin – in comparison to brown or black skin
- broken capillaries
- blue or red veins
- a proneness to prematurely ageing more quickly than other skins.

White skins vary between very fair to dark:

- fair and ruddy skins have warm undertones – beige and pinks
- ivory to fair skins have a light base with a hint of yellow undertone
- neutral fair skin would have no obvious undertone – just a beige undertone
- sallow skin may appear grey and have yellow undertones
- dark skin may be dark because of tanning and may have yellow or red undertones, depending upon its original tone.

Brown skins vary between fair and very dark:

- ivory to fair – having a warm beige undertone
- fair brown skin has a beige tone with a hint of yellow undertone
- mid-range brown skin has yellow undertones
- dark brown skin has yellow, orange and gold undertones
- the darkest of brown skins has gold, coral and orange undertones
- Armenian and Iranian skins, generally, have light to dark natural coral (orange) tones.

There is a great deal of variance in the tone of Indian and Pakistani skin colour. For example, in certain provinces of Pakistan there are people who are much lighter in skin colour than some Europeans, and therefore fall into a very fair category with a beige to pink undertone. However, in certain regions of India such as Calcutta, Madras and Goa the people, generally, have a much darker skin colour, similar to light black skin tones.

Black skins vary between light black and dark black:

- light black – yellow undertone
- medium black – yellow to gold undertone
- black – brown to orange undertone
- dark black – orange to red undertone *or* gold to olive undertone
- Afro-American – yellow to green in their native skin colour.

Black skins are the most unique as they do not age as fast as most other skins, this is because they have many more layers of **epidermal tissue** than fair skin and can withstand 'stress' for much longer.

Darker tones of foundation have a much higher pigment level, and a cream based foundation gives a much better coverage to the skin than liquid based foundation. This is because liquid foundations tend to be water based and therefore appear more translucent, whereas cream foundations are water and oil based and appear more opaque.

Ash coloured skin is a term used to describe a **keratinised** dehydrated condition that gives the skin a greyish appearance. Fair skin can have this same condition, but because of the lack of darker pigmentation it is not as apparent. Ashen skin can exist with all skin types: normal, combination, oily and – most commonly – dry.

1.5 Matching colours

Select three foundation colours – one light, one medium and one dark. Using red, yellow, blue, black and white paints, try to match them exactly.

Corrections to skin colour

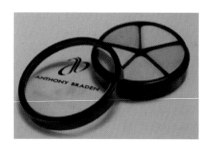

Neutralising wheel

You can correct most skin undertones by applying a small amount of its complementary colour. For example, for red or flushed skin or skin with broken capillaries, you can apply a small amount of green make-up concealer underneath the foundation. Yellow undertones can be minimised by the use of purple concealer applied underneath the foundation.

Although not a complementary colour, a blue **neutraliser** will counteract the grey ashy appearance some Asian skins have, with a foundation that matches the skin colour applied over it.

An orange or coral is useful for applying to dark shadows under the eyes on people from India and Pakistan. The orange/coral will take away the blue-black appearance of the shadow without making it look grey.

THE INFLUENCE OF LIGHTING ON MAKE-UP

Make-up varies with the surrounding circumstances and the existing light. In photography situations the most basic requirement of the lighting is to provide sufficient light to expose pictures in the camera, but lighting can also influence shape, depth, the character in the scene, atmosphere, composition and can direct the eye to a particular part of the scene. Skilful use of light on a face can accentuate or minimise the good or the bad features of the person being photographed.

It is essential that lighting and make-up work closely together. A lighting director will take into consideration all the shadows his or her lights will produce and aspects such as reflections in spectacles and contact lenses, while the make-up department corrects the smaller imperfections.

The overall aim of any documentary type production, whether it is TV, films or photography, is to achieve pictures that are sympathetic to the subject and comfortable to look at. In the case of a horror film, the overall aim is different, but the make-up and lighting would still need to be synchronised to make the most of the character. The lighting director will have responsibility for all lighting, but it is important for make-up, hair and costume staff to understand the principles of lighting to enable them to recognise if there is anything they can do to enhance a picture.

The main types of lighting used in film and photography work are as follows:

- *Key lights* – strong directional lights giving modelling and structure to a shot. The mood of the picture can be determined by how much light they produce – high key or low key.
- *Fill lights* – a softer source of light, often placed on the opposite side to the key light. They can be moved around easily and may have flaps on each side, called 'barn doors', which can be closed or opened to narrow or widen the effects. Coloured gels can be clipped to these lights to create different effects. Fill lights are extremely important when lighting faces.
- *Backlights* – sometimes a feeling of space between the artist and the background is required, and a light directed behind the subject will highlight the head.
- *Background lights* – give sufficient light to the background without over-powering the foreground.

Lighting and make-up

Top lighting will create shadows underneath any bone structure. Particularly difficult shadow areas are:

- under the eyebrows
- bags or lines under the eyes
- nose to mouth lines
- hollow cheeks
- under the chin.

Top lighting will also highlight the top of the head but cause heavy shadows under fringes and at the side of the face and neck if the model has long hair.

Studio lighting

If the studio has a make-up room, the lights around mirrors should be compatible with the lighting in the studio. Different bulbs, especially fluorescent bulbs, have different colour temperatures. If the bulbs are too orange, they will affect the make-up colours chosen, which will then not look right in the studio. Some fluorescent tubes have cooler colours resembling daylight. Unfortunately not all dressing rooms have good lighting and inadequate lighting will affect the work you do.

Flash testing

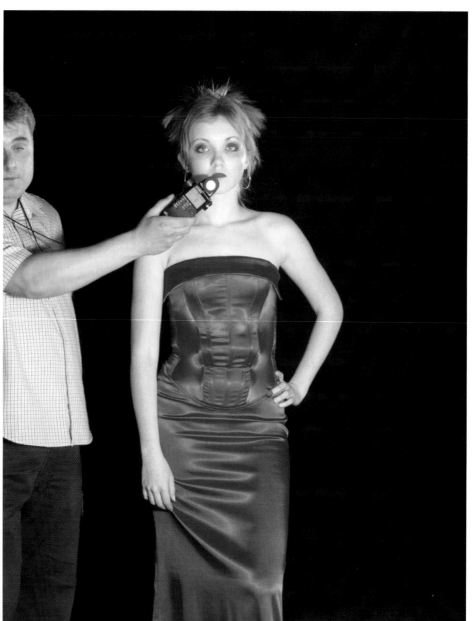

The photographer is using a special light meter to measure both the ambient light and the added effect of the flash head being used to illuminate the subject. Having measured the amount of light, he will know how to adjust either the flash power or the camera to get the required exposure.

Location lighting

It is especially important that make-up, hair and costume staff check their work in daylight when working out of doors, and keep continuity sheets. Even when performers or models are working outdoors, the make-up will have probably been done indoors. Often when filming out of doors in the daytime, minimal lighting is used – however scenes are often broken up into several sequences, and filmed out of sequence to be put together later, making careful note taking essential.

Assessment of knowledge and understanding

Knowledge review

1 What is the difference between light colour and pigment colour?

2 What would happen if you mixed all three primary pigment colours equally?

3 Give a definition of primary colours.

4 How do you make tints and shades?

5 What is brightness?

6 What is saturation?

7 What is harmony and contrast?

8 What colour would you use to correct a red flushed face?

9 What colour would you use to correct yellow undertones on a face?

10 What are, traditionally, the three primary pigment colours?

11 How would you describe secondary colours?

12 Colours can be described as warm or cool. Give two examples of each.

13 What are tertiary colours?

14 What are complementary colours?

15 How would you counteract an ashen skin tone?

16 What are fill lights?

17   What would top lighting do to a face?

18 What is the overall aim of lighting in any production, whether it is TV, films or photography?

19 What is a light meter used for?

20 What lighting would a photographer use if he wanted to create a feeling of space between the artist and the background?

chapter 2

Health and safety

Whatever area of make-up you work in, and wherever you are working, be it in a beauty salon, a TV studio, outside on a film set, or at a busy fashion show event, health and safety matters are of the utmost importance at all times. It is the responsibility of the make-up artist to maintain a safe, healthy and hygienic working environment to safeguard themselves, colleagues and models from accident and infection.

Learning objectives

In this chapter you will learn about:

- **achieving a professional appearance**
- **COSHH**
- **working safely**
- **working hygienically**
- **working efficiently**
- **kit boxes**

PROFESSIONAL APPEARANCE

It is necessary to maintain a high level of personal hygiene at all times. Remember the following golden rules:

- Keep your breath fresh with mints and mouthwash – especially important if you smoke or like garlic!
- Keep long hair tied back off the face.
- Keep your nails short and neatly manicured – long fingernails can be dangerous.
- Be minimal with your own make-up during working hours.

- Wear comfortable flat shoes – high heels are dangerous around TV studios, film sets and general working places.
- Keep deodorant wipes handy – you will be working very close to models, and there is nothing worse than stale body odour.

CONTROL OF SUBSTANCES HAZARDOUS TO HEALTH (COSHH) 2002

The COSHH 2002 regulations provide guidance and lay down rules about the safe storage and use of potentially dangerous substances. You should be familiar with these regulations, a copy of which can be obtained from your learning establishment or the office of your local Health & Safety Executive (HSE). In particular you should know the correct way to store and use cleaning agents and how to ensure that the storage area is clearly identified.

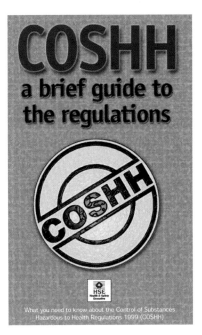

COSHH regulation booklet

WORKING SAFELY

- Make-up products should always be labelled clearly, with full instructions for use if applicable. This is to avoid accidents such as mistaking surgical spirit or acetone for a skin toner.
- Hazardous materials should be kept securely in lockable cabinets or metal trunks.
- Electrical sockets, plugs and electric equipment (like hair-dryers) must be checked regularly. Any equipment which has frayed wires or is faulty must not be used and must be replaced or repaired immediately.
- Solvent removers must be disposed of safely in covered bins.
- Make-up work must always be undertaken in a well-ventilated area.

WORKING HYGIENICALLY

- Towels, hair bands and protective gowns must always be clean and freshly laundered.
- Wherever you are working, there should be a washbasin with hot and cold running water.
- In case there is no running water, always carry a hand sanitiser in your kit box.
- Tools and equipment must be sterilised. Clean electrical equipment such as shavers, beard trimmers and tongs with surgical spirit.
- Mirrors should be kept polished.

- Check that all powder puffs, brushes, sponges, etc. are cleaned thoroughly immediately after a make-up application, and always before each new model. If working on multiple models throughout the day, clean these items between models, or use disposable items whenever possible.

- Never use lipsticks, or other make-up products directly from the container to the model's face. Always use a spatula to transfer the product onto a palette. There are many types available, including plastic and stainless steel. Take care if using a ceramic tile, as these break easily. From the palette use either a new disposable brush or an appropriate clean brush to apply the product.

WORKING EFFICIENTLY

Do not run out of product. If you are freelance, you alone are responsible for not running out of products. If you are an employee and you see a product coming to an end, or you take the last one from a stock cupboard, report any needs to the production office, the supervisor, or whoever is responsible for re-ordering stock – but do not wait until the product has completely run out.

Planning ahead

Whether a big wedding party is coming into the salon, or you are going on location, it is essential to plan ahead. This should cover everything – your make-up kit, continuity reference materials from previously made-up models, models for this job, actors, and your personal effects – including your passport if you are going on location abroad – together with sensible and appropriate clothing. If you are freelance, you will need to know the exact address of the location at which you will be working – and leave in plenty of time to get there. Double check dates and arrangements. The end result will be a calm and well-organised make-up artist – the type that is offered more work!

KIT BOXES

Products

Your make-up kit boxes should be well-organised and clean at all times. Absolutely no excuses! Keep your fashion make-up and theatrical/film make-up in separate boxes. If it is not obvious what an item is, then label it. Organise your kit box in such a way that nothing will get damaged, split or broken. Anything potentially messy, such as artificial blood or **glycerine**, should be stored separately, wrapped in plastic bags, or cling film if necessary. Always keep any 'glitter' products totally separate from all other make-up – together with the brushes you use to apply them. Plastic containers are preferable to glass ones for safety reasons, but double check before decanting anything that the product can in fact be stored in plastic bottles – for example surgical spirit, isopropyl alcohol and cleaning solvents must be kept in glass containers. When models or potential employers see a dirty, messy and disorganised make-up box, they will assume the standard of your work will be the same – dirty, messy and disorganised!!

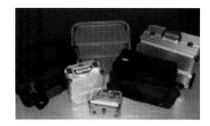

Equipment

Your brushes, sponges and powder puffs are the tools of your trade. They should be obviously clean and well-organised.

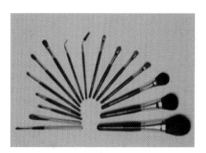

Brushes

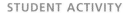

STUDENT ACTIVITY

2.1 Health and Safety and your kit box

Go through your make-up kit box, and with the help of your colleagues and lecturer, list everything that might be described as a potentially dangerous substance. Identify any products that are not suitable for storage in plastic bottles.

Assessment of knowledge and understanding

Knowledge review

1 Name four activities you can do to achieve a professional appearance.

2 What does COSHH stand for?

3 What do the COSHH regulations provide?

4 What steps can you take to ensure your working environment is a safe place to work?

5 How should you hygienically use a lipstick?

6 What steps can you take to work efficiently?

7 How can you organise your kit box so you can find items easily?

8 What can you do if there is no running water where you are working?

9 What products, in particular, should be stored separately in your make-up kit box?

10 What type of products cannot be stored in plastic bottles?

chapter 3

Anatomy and physiology

It is imperative for all make-up artists to have a good understanding of the related anatomy and physiology involved when working on a model's face. Not only is knowledge of the bone structure of the human skull necessary, the formation of facial muscles and an in-depth knowledge of the skin are also important. This related anatomy and physiology will enable you to identify infectious and non-infectious skin diseases and to become aware of abnormal looking moles and skin conditions. Learning the facial muscles of expression will help you with the practical make-up application of highlighting and shading in the correct areas for the desired result. You will also be able to perform facial massage without causing any discomfort.

Learning objectives

In this chapter you will learn about:

- the bones of the head and face
- the muscles that allow us to create facial expressions
- the structure and functions of the skin
- infectious and non-infectious skin diseases
- sun-damaged skin and sunscreens
- moles and skin cancers
- skin types
- how the natural ageing process affects skin

BONES OF THE HEAD AND FACE

The skeleton gives the body shape. It also provides attachment for the muscles and protects delicate organs; the skull for example protects the brain. To aid good make-up application, the make-up artist should have an understanding of the main bones of the head and face.

Bones that form the skull

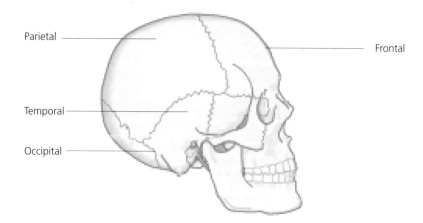

Bones that form the face

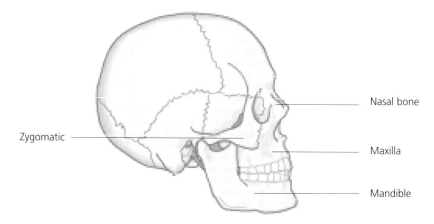

The bones that form the head are collectively known as the skull. The skull can be divided into two parts, the face and the cranium.

Bones of the skull

Bone	Position and function
Occipital × 1	The lower back of the skull. Contains a large hole called the *foramen magnum*, through which passes the spinal cord, nerves and blood vessels.
Parietal × 2	Positioned at the back and sides of the head forming the roof of the skull – commonly called 'the crown'.
Frontal × 1	Forms the front of the skull, forehead and upper eye sockets.
Temporal × 2	Either side of the head, around the ears, providing important muscle attachment points for the **mastoid process** and the **zygomatic process**.

Bones of the face

Bone	Position and function
Zygomatic × 2	These form the cheek bones.
Maxilla × 2	Fused together to form the upper jaw, which holds the upper teeth.
Mandible × 1	The largest and strongest of the facial bones holding the lower teeth. It is the only moving bone in the face allowing movement of the mouth for chewing and talking.
Nasal × 2	Forms the bridge of the nose.

MUSCLES OF FACIAL EXPRESSION AND MASTICATION

Many of the muscles located in the face are very small and are either attached to other small muscles or attached directly to the facial skin. When the muscles contract, they pull the facial skin in a particular way and it is these continuous movements that create facial expression. It is the movements of some of these muscles that allows us to chew our food – known as **mastication**.

With age, the facial expressions we make every day produce lines on the skin – frown lines, smile lines and laughter lines. An understanding of the position, functions and facial expressions of these muscles will enable you to be more creative in all your make-up work, especially character work. You may need to insert facial expression lines that are absent from a model to make the face look older, sad or happy.

STUDENT ACTIVITY

3.1 Muscles of the face
Pleasant and sombre expressions

As you colour in each muscle, try locating it on yourself while looking into a mirror. Locate the muscle on both sides of the face and note the difference.

1 Colour the muscles creating the pleasant expression on the left side, using bright warm and cheerful colours. Colour only the lettered muscles.

2 Do the same on the right side using sombre bluish colours.

3 Colour the remaining facial muscles in grey.

4 Colour the major muscles of mastication a neutral colour.

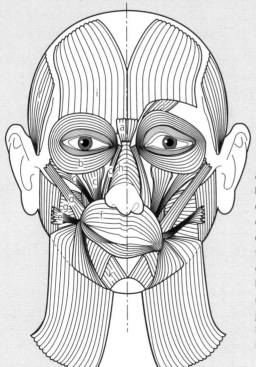

a. procerus
b. orbicularis oculi
c. quadratus labii superioris
d. zygomaticus major
e. risorius
f. orbicularis oris
g. buccinator
h. nasalis
i. frontalis
j. corrugator
k. mentalis
l. temporalis masseter

Muscles of the face

Muscle	Position, function and expression
Frontalis	The forehead – upper part of the cranium. The scalp moves forward, raises the eyebrows and gives an expression of surprise.
Corrugator	Between the eyebrows – draws the eyebrows together, giving an expression of frowning.
Procerus	Top of the nose between the eyebrows – depresses the eyebrows, making wrinkles over the bridge of the nose.
Orbicularis Oculi	Surrounds the eye and closes the eyelids – used in blinking and winking.
Nasalis	Over the front of the nose – compresses the nose causing wrinkles.
Temporalis	Runs down side of face towards upper jaw – aids chewing and closing the mouth.
Masseter	Runs down the back to the angle of the jaw – lifts the jaw and gives the teeth strength for biting.
Buccinator	Inside the cheeks, giving form and shape – puffs out cheeks when blowing and keeps food in mouth when chewing.
Risorius	In the lower cheek, extending diagonally from the corners of the mouth – they draw the corners of the mouth outwards and give an expression of smiling.
Zygomaticus Major	Runs down the cheek towards the corner of the mouth – pulls the corner of the mouth upwards and sideways as in smiling and laughing.
Orbicularis oris	Surrounds the lips and forms the mouth – purses the lip, closes the mouth and gives the expressions of pouting and kissing.
Triangularis	Corner of the lower lip, extends over the chin – this muscle draws down the mouth's corners giving an expression of sadness.
Mentalis	Forms the chin, raises the lower lip, causing the chin to wrinkle and giving an expression of doubt.
Quadratus labii superiorus	Runs upwards from the upper lip – lifts the upper lip and helps to open the mouth.

STRUCTURE AND FUNCTIONS OF THE SKIN

The human skin is an organ – the largest of the body. It provides a tough, flexible covering, with many important functions.

As make-up artists you will be working with skin every day. You will be covering the face and neck and, on occasion, other parts of the body not only with make-up products, but adhesives, sequins, glitter, paints, **prosthetics** or **postiche**, so it is important you check with models, *prior* to application for any known sensitivities they have to products. You need to encourage skin tests for new products, especially adhesives and face paints used on children, and you need to be able to identify any abnormal reactions models may have to products. It is also important for you to be able to identify skin diseases – infectious and non-infectious – and be able to give advice on how to look after the skin in general. You also need an awareness of moles and skin cancers and the guidelines for protection.

Structure

The skin has three main distinct layers: the **epidermis**, the **dermis** and the **subcutaneous** layers. Between these layers is a specialised layer which acts like a 'glue', sticking the layers together; this is the **basement membrane**. If the epidermis and dermis become separated, body fluids fill the space, creating a blister. The subcutaneous layer is situated below the epidermis and dermis and is often called the fat layer. It is this layer that provides protection to the underlying organs.

The epidermis

The epidermis is the outermost layer of the skin. It is made up of five layers:

1 Horny layer (Stratum corneum)
2 Clear layer (Stratum lucidium)
3 Granular layer (Stratum granulosum)
4 Prickle cell layer (Stratum spinosum)
5 Basal cell layer (Stratum germativum)

Horny layer

This is the most superficial, outer layer, consisting of dead, flattened, keratinised cells which have taken approximately a month to travel from the germinating layer. This outer layer of dead cells is continually being shed in a process known as **desquamation**.

Clear layer

This layer consists of transparent cells that permit light to pass through. It comprises three or four rows of flat dead cells that are completely filled with keratin; they have no **nuclei** as the cells have undergone **mitosis**. The clear layer is very shallow in facial skin but much thicker on the soles of the feet and palms of the hands, while it is generally absent in hairy skin.

Granular layer

This layer consists of distinctly shaped cells, containing a number of granules, which are involved in the hardening of the cells by the process of keratinisation. This layer links the living cells of the epidermis to the dead cells above.

Prickle cell layer

This is known as the prickle cell layer because each of the rounded cells contained within it has short projections that make contact with the neighbouring cells and give them a prickly appearance. The living cells of this layer are capable of dividing by the process of mitosis.

Basal cell layer

This is the deepest of the five layers. It consists of a single layer of column cells on a basement membrane that separates the epidermis from the dermis. In this layer, the new epidermal cells are constantly being reproduced. These cells last about six weeks from reproduction or mitosis before being discarded into the horny layer. New cells are therefore formed by division, pushing adjacent cells towards the skin's surface. At intervals between the column cells, which divide to reproduce, are the large star-shaped cells called melanocytes, which form the pigment **melanin**, the skin's main colouring agent.

The dermis

The dermis is the inner portion of the skin, situated underneath the epidermis and composed of dense **connective tissue**. It is often referred to as the 'true' skin because it contains the main components of the skin such as nerve endings (for sensitivity to pain, pressure, hot, cold, etc.), the blood supply and the lymph vessels, hair follicles and our sweat glands for temperature regulation. The dermis is much thicker than the epidermis. The key functions of the dermis are to provide support, strength and elasticity. The dermis has a superficial papillary layer and a deep reticular layer.

The papillary layer

The superficial **papillary layer** is made up of adipose (fatty) connective tissue and is connected to the underside of the epidermis by tiny cone-shaped projections called papillae; these contain both nerve endings and blood capillaries. The papillary layer also supplies the upper epidermis with its nutrition.

The reticular layer

The dermis contains a network of protein fibres called the **reticular layer**. These fibres allow the skin to expand, contract, and perform intricate, supple movements. This network is composed of three sorts of protein fibre: yellow elastin fibres, white collagen fibres and reticular fibres. Elastin fibres give the skin its elasticity, collagen fibres give it strength, and reticular fibres help to support and hold all the structures in place. All these fibres help maintain the skin's *tone* (in this context, this word does not have the same meaning as it did in the discussion of colour in Chapter 1; here it refers to firmness and suppleness). The fibres are produced by specialised cells called fibroblasts, and are held in a gel called the ground substance.

While this network is strong, the skin will appear youthful and firm. As the fibres harden and fragment, however, the network begins to collapse, losing its elasticity. The skin then begins to show visible signs of ageing.

The subcutaneous tissue

This is the fatty layer of the skin, situated underneath the dermis. Cells called lipocytes produce lipids, which are the fat cells from which we form subcutaneous tissue. The function of the subcutaneous layer is to protect the muscles, bones and internal organs from being damaged and to provide insulation against the cold. It also provides a source of energy if the body should need it.

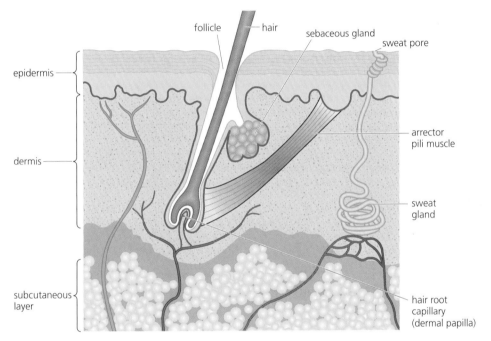

The structure of the skin

Other structures in the skin

A number of other structures are also found in the dermis and subcutaneous layers of the skin:

- *Blood vessels* consist of arteries, veins and capillaries. Arteries carry nutrients and oxygen to the skin via the capillaries. Veins remove waste products. Capillaries also help with heat regulation.
- *Nerves*. Sensory nerve endings can be found on the dermis and subcutaneous tissue. These nerve endings respond to pain, pressure, heat, cold and touch. The nerves carry impulses to the brain for responses by the body for protection or action.
- *Arector pili muscles* can be found within muscle tissue. They are attached to the hair follicle at the base of the epidermis. Their function is to raise the hair follicle to close the pore and so trap warmth in the body.

- *Sebaceous glands* are found in the dermis, adjacent to hair follicles. They produce sebum to lubricate the hair and the skin. Sebum combines with sweat to form the acid mantle; this helps to waterproof the skin.
- *Hair* grows in the follicles in the dermis and is then seen growing out through the epidermis. Believed to be connected to the production of body warmth. It is also a gender characteristic. Hair is not present on the soles of the feet and the palms of the hand or on the lips.
- *Hair follicle* – a threadlike outgrowth of the epidermis. Found in the dermis but not present on the soles of the feet or the palms of the hands or lips. Hair follicles produce and contain the hair during its life cycle.
- *Sudoriferous glands*
  - *sweat glands* are known as eccrine glands. Eccrine glands are found all over the body but are dense on the palms of the hands and soles of the feet. These glands produce sweat, water and **urea**, so help to regulate body temperature, remove **toxin** accumulations and contribute to the acid mantle.
  - *apocrine glands* – these are fewer in number and larger than eccrine glands. They are only found in hairy parts of the body, that is the armpits, nipples, anal and genital areas. Apocrine glands are under the control of the nervous system and respond to sexual attraction, emotional demands and psychological factors.

INFECTIOUS AND NON-INFECTIOUS DISEASES OF THE SKIN

It is important that a make-up treatment is not carried out if any contra indication is present. **Contra indications** include:

- bacterial/viral and fungal infections of eyes, lips or face
- open cuts and abrasions
- broken bones
- acute acne
- severe eczema or psoriasis

The following conditions are contra indicated to make-up application on the face. It is your responsibility as a make-up artist to protect yourself and future models from contamination via these micro-organisms. No matter how well you may wash your hands, brushes and equipment, they will still be infected and you may pass it on to someone else. Abstain from applying make-up to someone if they have any of these infectious diseases.

TIP	

Real Life Situation! There may be occasions when you simply have to make-up someone with one of these conditions, a news presenter going on air, an actress or actor on the final day of shooting, etc. If there is no alternative, then you must protect yourself – wear disposable gloves, wear a disposable mask, use disposable brushes and avoid the affected area totally if you can. If the model has a cold sore on the lips, concentrate on great eye make-up and hair styling, emphasising these areas and avoiding the cold sore. Keep these disposable protective items in your make-up box, in case of emergency.

Bacterial infections

Impetigo

Highly infectious, this starts as small red spots, which then break open and form blisters. Most common around the corner of the mouth and if picked will spread. Can be spread through the use of dirty equipment.

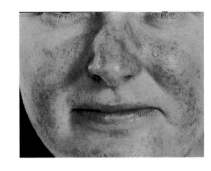

Impetigo

Boils

This infection forms at the base of a hair follicle. Bacteria can spread through an open scratch in the skin. The area is raised, red and painful. Pus may be present.

Conjunctivitis

This is a nasty eye condition. The eyelids are red and sore, with itching. Mainly caused by bacteria being present; it can be irritated by a virus or an allergy.

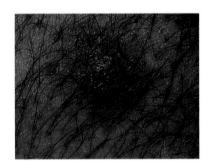

Boils

Stye

This is a small boil at the base of the eyelash follicle. It is raised, sore and red, and there may be considerable swelling in the area.

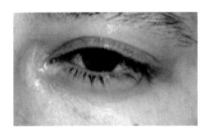

Conjunctivitis

Fungal infections

Ringworm

Red pimples appear and then form a circle, with clear skin in the middle. It is highly contagious and scales and pustules follow. It can be spread onto the face from any other area of the body. It can be passed onto humans by contact with domestic animals.

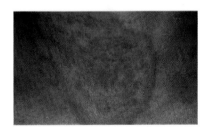

Ringworm

Blepharitis

An infection of the eye lid causing inflammation; the eye will look red and sore. Depending on the severity of the condition, it may be better to avoid eye make-up application altogether, and focus attention on the mouth, with a pretty lipstick shade.

Viruses

The common cold

Freely recognised. Streaming eyes and nose, coughing and sneezing that is easily spread.

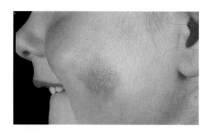

Cold Sore

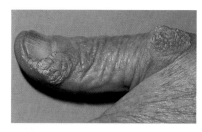

Warts

Cold sores

Found on the lips, cheeks and nose. Blisters form, the skin is broken and painful; the blisters are especially likely to spread when open and weepy and then crusts form.

Warts

Small compact raised growths of skin – can be light or brown in colour, present on the face and neck. Warts on the hand are the same as veruccas on the feet – highly contagious.

Non-infectious skin conditions

The following conditions are not infections, so a make-up application can take place but may need some adaptation.

Acne vulgaris

Oily skin, papules, pustules, cysts and scars describes the appearance of acne vulgaris. Mostly associated with hormones, the condition is common among adolescents. The presence of bacteria can make the condition infected and therefore contra indicated for a make-up treatment. However, a model with mild acne can be worked upon.

Acne rosacea

Flushing of cheeks and nose, dilated capillaries, progresses to papules, pustules and scales. The cause is largely unknown although factors such as spicy food, alcohol, heat, menopause and emotional stress may be contributory. The application of a neutralising colour of make-up can tone down the redness and therefore lessen the 'angry' look of the skin.

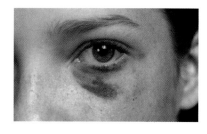

Bruising

Bruising

Avoid bruised areas altogether if recent and painful to touch. If the area is turning yellow, showing that healing is taking place, then a gentle application of make-up will help to blend in the colour differences to the model's normal skin shade.

Cuts and abrasions

Open cuts should be covered and the area avoided altogether. An old cut that has healed over and is not too sore can have make-up applied gently, whilst carefully considering all hygiene matters.

Dermatitis

An inflammation of the skin, where skin appears red and dry. Often caused by the skin having contact with external irritants. The skin's appearance is similar to eczema in appearance, but the cause is not the same. Use hypo-allergenic make-up or ask the model if they would prefer you to use their own make-up.

Eczema

Patches of very dry, red skin which appear cracked and scaly and are often itchy. Hypo-allergenic products are recommended for dry eczema. There is also a condition where the skin may weep, known as wet eczema. Wet eczema is contra indicated and should not have make-up applied to it.

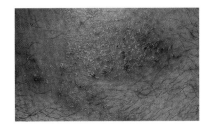

Eczema

Milia

These are small white lumps under the skin, often around the eyes or on the side of the cheek, caused by a build-up of sebum. Make-up application can take place over milia, as they are not infectious.

Psoriasis

Red plaques of skin covered by white, silvery scales; affects all parts of the body but particularly elbows and knees. Psoriasis can also affect the nails and be found in the scalp. Caused by faulty keratinisation of skin. Stress is often an aggravating factor.

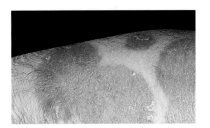

Psoriasis

Scar tissue

Scar tissue less than six months old should not be touched with make-up as the healing process is still taking place. If the scar is healing, and over six months old, then a gentle application of a camouflage make-up can be used with the model's permission.

Skin tags

Usually found on the eye area or lids and/or on the side of the neck. Often found in more elderly models. They are not infectious or painful and make-up application can take place. They can easily be removed by a GP under local anaesthetic.

Pigmentation disorders

Caused by irregularities in the skin's melanin production. They are not infectious and not contra indicated to make-up application. Conditions such as vitiligo, chloasma, port wine stains and many others are discussed in detail in Chapter 12 'Camouflage make-up'.

SUN DAMAGED SKIN AND SUNSCREENS

Too much exposure to the sun can cause significant damage to human skin. Over time, the sun's heat tends to dry out areas of unprotected skin and to deplete the skin's supply of natural lubricating oils. In addition the sun's ultraviolet (UV) radiation can cause both short-term burning and long-term changes in the skin's structure.

The most common types of damage to the skin from the sun are:

- dry skin
- sunburn
- actinic keratosis
- photo-ageing and senile purpura

These problems can be recognised by the following symptoms:

- *Dry skin* – sun-exposed skin can gradually lose moisture and essential oils, making it appear dry, flaky and prematurely wrinkled.
- *Sunburn* – sunburn is the common name for the short-term skin damage caused by UV radiation. Mild sunburn causes painful reddening of the skin, but more severe cases can produce tiny fluid-filled bumps (vesicles) or larger blisters.
- *Actinic keratosis* – this is a small, scaly patch of sun-damaged skin that has a pink, red, yellow or brownish tint. Unlike suntan markings or sunburns, an actinic keratosis does not go away. It develops in areas of skin that have undergone repeated or long-term exposure to the sun's UV light, and it is a warning sign of an increased risk of skin cancer.
- *Photo-ageing* and *senile purpura* are phrases used to describe long-term changes in the skin's collagen. With photo-ageing, the skin develops wrinkles and fine lines because of UV-related changes in the collagen of the dermis. In senile purpura, UV radiation damages the **structural collagen** that supports the walls of the skin's tiny blood vessels. This makes blood vessels more fragile and more liable to bruising.

Over a lifetime, repeated episodes of sunburn and unprotected sun exposure can also increase a person's risk of skin cancer. As a rule, if you have fair skin and light eyes, you are at greater risk of sun-related skin damage and skin cancers. This is because your skin contains less melanin, which helps to protect the skin from the effects of UV radiation.

In most cases a doctor can confirm sun-damaged skin simply by examining the area. Sometimes a **biopsy** may be necessary to rule out skin cancer in a patch of actinic keratosis.

The painful redness of sunburn tends to fade within a few days, provided the injured skin is not re-exposed to the sun without using a sun block or sunscreen. Other forms of sun damage tend to be long-term conditions, although prescription medications, non-prescription remedies and skin-resurfacing treatments may improve the skin's appearance.

The treatment required depends on the form of sun damage:

- *Dry skin* – use a body lotion regularly; avoid taking hot baths or hot showers as these can make your sun-damaged skin even drier. Wash only with warm or cool water, using soap that either has a high fat content or contains glycerin.
- *Sunburn* – for painful sunburn, apply cool compresses to the injured skin, or mist the area with sprays of cool water. If the discomfort continues, visit a doctor who may prescribe anti-inflammatory medication if there is extensive sunburn with severe blistering and pain.
- **Actinic keratosis** – the type of treatment that will work best for you depends on many factors including the number, size and location of the patches of actinic keratosis. The range of options includes:
  - watchful waiting – there is no immediate treatment, but the doctor regularly monitors the area of abnormal skin
  - topical medication – an anti-cancer drug is applied directly to the skin to eliminate the actinic keratosis
  - cryosurgery – the actinic keratosis is frozen with liquid nitrogen
  - chemical peels – a strong chemical solution is used to remove the top layer of skin, which later re-grows
  - laser resurfacing – this works in the same way as a chemical peel, but it uses a laser beam instead of a chemical solution
  - shave excision – a doctor carefully shaves away the area of abnormal skin. If necessary, the skin shavings can be used as a biopsy specimen to check for cancer.
- **Photo-ageing** and other collagen changes – although it is not possible to reverse all of the effects of long-term sun damage, doctors can sometimes improve the appearance of skin by prescribing treatments in the form of vitamin A derivatives, or strong alpha-hydroxy acids that are applied directly to the skin.

Cosmetically, the prognosis is excellent for most skin problems resulting from sun exposure. Most treatments for an actinic keratosis can leave a pale (de-pigmented) area of the skin surface. More important than appearance, however, is the long-term impact of sun damage on your chances of developing skin cancer. Overall the greater amount of unprotected sun exposure you have during your lifetime, the greater your risk of skin cancer, especially if you have a light complexion.

HEALTH AND SAFETY

Always seek your doctor's advice if you notice any abnormal changes in your skin's appearance.

MOLES AND SKIN CANCERS

Moles

Moles are spots on the skin – nearly everyone has them. In fact, babies are born with moles that are flesh colour and through time they enlarge and darken, making them more noticeable.

Moles occur when skin cells called melanocytes grow in clusters, instead of being spread evenly throughout the skin. Melanocytes make the pigment melanin that gives skin its natural colour. Melanin darkens under ultraviolet (UV) light from the sun or tanning beds and creates a tan.

A single mole is called 'naevus' and multiple moles are called 'naevi'.

What does a normal mole look like?

All the following mole varieties are considered perfectly safe:

- Normal moles are evenly coloured and may or may not be raised. They have clear, even edges, and are usually circular or oval in shape.
- Normal freckles are simply coloured spots and can range in size from 1 to 10 mm.
- Seborrhoeic keratoses are common in older people with a history of sun exposure. They have a very discrete edge and often sit up on top of the skin. Colours vary from pale skin to orange and black.

Melanoma warning signs

The warning signs of the possible presence of melanoma in a mole include:

- **A**symmetry – the mole looses symmetry and its normal circular or oval shape
- **B**order – the mole outline becomes irregular
- **C**olour – the mole develops more than one colour or shade
- **D**iameter – the mole becomes greater than 5 mm in size, i.e. the width of a pencil

If people detect a mole with these features, it is important to seek advice. However, people should not assume the absence of such features means a mole is melanoma free. There are now Advanced Mole Screening systems available which evaluate all these features (see The Mole Clinic in the list of resources at the end of the book). Clients receive a graphic print out of their results, confirming whether or not a mole should be removed. Virtually all melanoma – or the absence of melanoma – is instantly and automatically confirmed. If a medium to high risk of melanoma is identified, clients are referred to their GP or a consultant surgeon specialising in skin cancer for advice and treatment. Moles with a low risk of melanoma are reviewed at a later date and any changes identified. Anyone facing the removal of a suspect mole can now have that mole analysed and, if confirmed melanoma-free, can often avoid that removal.

Are abnormal moles common?

Around 1 in 10 people have at least one abnormal mole – *dysplastic naevi* – on their body. Recent studies reveal that they are more likely to turn into melanoma than normal moles. Not everyone who has abnormal moles develop melanoma. Most moles, both normal and abnormal, never turn cancerous. It is important, however, to keep abnormal moles under review and to be able to recognise the warning signs.

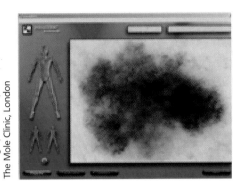
Melanoma mole

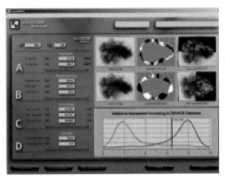
Melanoma mole scored

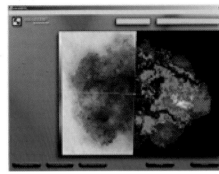
Melanoma mole analysed

Risk factors for sun-damaged skin, non-melanoma and melanoma skin cancers

- *Sun exposure* – the single greatest risk factor for most skin cancers is unprotected exposure to the sun's ultraviolet rays.

- *Gender and age* – men have twice the rate of basal-cell **carcinoma** and three times the rate of squamous-cell carcinoma as women, perhaps because of outdoor occupations that expose them to the sun. The risk of basal and squamous-cell cancers increases with age.

- *Fair skin* – the risk of skin cancer is more than 20 times higher for white-skinned than for dark-skinned people. Those with fair skin with freckles or who burn easily face the highest risk. This is because darker skin has more skin pigment, which offers a protective effect against the sun's UV rays.

- *Radiation exposure* – people who have had radiation treatment have a greater risk of developing non-melanoma skin cancer in the area that was treated. This risk begins about 20 years after the radiation treatment.

- *Reduced immunity* – people with weakened immune systems are more likely to develop non-melanoma skin cancer. This includes individuals with HIV infection and organ transplant recipients, who are usually given medications that suppress their immune system to prevent their body from rejecting the new organ.

- *Chemical exposure* – exposure to industrial tar, coal and some types of oil can increase the risk of squamous-cell cancer. Arsenic, a naturally occurring substance in rock formations and soil, is contained in wood preservatives and is a byproduct of brass and bronze manufacture, copper smelting and glass making. It can contaminate drinking water and has been associated with both types of non-melanoma skin cancer.

- *Genetic syndromes* – several rare inherited syndromes can predispose an individual to non-melanoma skin cancer including **albinism**, **nevoid basal-cell carcinoma syndrome**, **xeroderma pigmentosum** and **epidermodysplasia verruciformis**.

- *Injury and inflammation* – skin cancer can develop in ulcers, scars and other skin injuries that do not heal. There is a small risk of developing non-melanoma cancer in skin affected by skin diseases such as **discoid lupus erythematosus**.

Prevention

You can help prevent skin becoming sun-damaged and skin cancers by taking the following steps:

- Apply a sunscreen before you go outdoors. Choose a sunscreen that has a sun protection factor of 15 or above, with a broad spectrum of protection against both UV-A and UV-B rays.
- Use a sun block on your lips. Choose a product that has been specially formulated for the lips, with a sun protection factor of 20 or more.
- Limit your time outdoors when the sun is at its peak – between 12–2 in most European countries.
- Wear sunglasses with UV light protection – not as a fashion accessory.
- Wear light clothing that covers the arms and legs and a hat with a wide brim.
- Be aware that some medications and skin-care products can increase your skin's risk of UV damage. These include certain antibiotics, as well as some prescription medicines. If you are prescribed a medicine and you normally spend a great deal of time outdoors, ask your doctor whether you should take any special precautions to avoid sun exposure. Products containing alpha-hydroxy acids can also make your skin more vulnerable to damage from sunlight.
- Examine your entire skin surface thoroughly every month. Check for patches of discoloured or scaly skin, moles, small pearly nodules, sores and other skin abnormalities on all parts of your body. Use a mirror to inspect harder-to-see areas of your back, shoulders, upper arms, buttocks and the soles of your feet.
- Avoid sunbeds – if you need to appear tanned, use commercial sunless tanning creams and follow the manufacturer's instructions carefully.

Melanoma

In melanoma, melanocytes undergo cancerous changes and reproduce aggressively to form a life-threatening **tumour**. Melanoma is the deadliest form of skin cancer and is increasing at faster rates than any other cancer. It is now the most common cancer in the 15–39 age group. Last year, almost twice as many Britons died of melanoma than Australians. This is because Australians undergo frequent screening as routine.

Your risk of developing melanoma is higher if you have:

- red or blond hair, or green or blue eyes
- fair skin
- excessive sun exposure, especially in childhood
- a first-degree relative (mother, father, sister or brother) with melanoma – if you have a first-degree relative with melanoma, you are eight times more likely to develop melanoma yourself.

The following skin changes indicate an increased risk of melanoma:

- new mole appearing after the age of 30
- new mole at any age if it is in an area that is rarely exposed to the sun
- change in an existing mole.

- one or more dysplastic nevi, also called 'atypical moles' – a mole is given this distinction if it has any features that make it resemble a melanoma
- at least 20 moles greater than 2 mm in diameter
- at least 5 moles greater than 5 mm in diameter
- freckles caused by exposure to the sun

Unlike internal cancers, melanoma is visible on your skin making early detection easier. Melanoma can be cured if it is found and treated early when the tumor is small and has not penetrated deeply into the skin. More advanced melanoma require prolonged treatment and can be fatal.

Non-melanoma skin cancer

Non-melanoma skin cancers include basal-cell cancers, which account for 80 per cent of all skin cancers, and squamous-cell cancers, which account for 15 per cent of skin cancer cases.

Basal-cell cancers originate in the basal cells of the epidermis. They usually develop on areas of the body that have been exposed to the sun – the face, ears, neck, scalp, shoulders and back. Most cases are probably caused by ultraviolet B (UV-B) radiation. These slow-growing cancers rarely spread internally. People who have had one basal-cell carcinoma have a 35–50 per cent chance of developing a new one within five years, usually at another site that has been exposed to the sun.

Squamous-cell cancers occur in the epidermis and usually appear on sun-exposed surfaces of the body, like the face, ears, neck, lips, backs of the hands, arms, chest, the back and the legs. In rare cases, these cancers may develop in skin that has been damaged or diseased by a process other than sun exposure, for example in scars from severe burns, in skin ulcers and, less often, in the genital area. Genital squamous-cell cancers can arise as a result of a sexually transmitted infection with the human papilloma virus (a virus associated with genital warts and cervical cancer). Squamous-cell cancer is more aggressive than basal-cell carcinoma, with approximately 3 per cent of cases spreading to distant areas of the body.

SKIN TYPES

- caucasian skin
- dark skin

Caucasian skin

Caucasian skin types are usually described in one of four ways:

1 normal

2 dry

3 oily

4 combination

In addition to these four basic categories, there may also be additional characteristics. The skin may also be:

- sensitive
- dehydrated
- mature

Identifying a true skin type is made more difficult by the fact there are many environmental and lifestyle factors that contribute to the condition of the skin. For example, too much sun exposure can cause significant damage to human skin, as already discussed in this chapter. Other factors include those discussed below.

Normal skin

Normal skin is an ideal skin type, but rare to find. It is often referred to as balanced because it is neither too dry nor too oily. Characteristics of a normal skin are:

- the skin texture is even, neither too thick nor too thin
- the skin has a healthy colour
- the skin elasticity is good; when you pinch the skin, it recoils immediately
- the skin feels firm to the touch
- the skin pigmentation is even-coloured
- the skin is usually free from blemishes

Dry skin

This type of skin is oil and/or moisture deficient, leaving the skin dry to the touch. There may be some loss of elasticity depending upon the model's age. Because sebum limits moisture loss by evaporation from the skin, skin with insufficient sebum rapidly loses moisture. The resulting dry skin is often described as dehydrated. Its characteristics include:

- the pores are small and tight
- the moisture content is poor
- the skin texture is coarse and thin, with patches of visibly flaking skin
- there is a tendency towards sensitivity (broken capillaries often accompany this skin type)
- premature ageing is common, resulting in the appearance of wrinkles, seen especially around the eyes, mouth and neck
- skin pigmentation may be uneven resulting in freckles
- milia are often found around the cheek and eye area

Oily skin

Oily or greasy skin is caused by an over-production of sebum from the sebaceous glands and can cause blemishes. This skin type is also referred to as seborrhoeic and it has the following characteristics:

- the pores are enlarged
- the moisture content is high
- the skin is coarse and thick
- the skin is sallow in colour, as a result of the excess sebum production, dead skin cells having become embedded in the sebum, and the skin having sluggish blood and lymph circulation
- the skin tone is good, due to the protective effect of the sebum
- the skin is prone to shininess, due to excess sebum production
- there may be uneven pigmentation
- certain skin disorders may be apparent – **comedones**, pustules, papules, milia or sebaceous cysts.

Combination skin

Some skins are a combination of two or more skin types and the most common one is a greasy T-zone along the forehead and nose, with normal or dry skin on the cheek area. This is because there are more sebaceous glands along the T-zone which may therefore show all the characteristics of greasy skin.

Additional characteristics

- *Sensitive* – a sensitive skin reacts easily to even mild stimulus – products or even touch. Often dry skins, lacking in sebum and therefore unprotected by it, are sensitive. Sensitive skins can have a highly flushed look, have a tendency to colour easily and can react to make-up and other products.
- *Dehydrated* – a dehydrated skin lacks moisture. The condition can affect any skin type, but most commonly accompanies dry or combination skin types. A dehydrated skin often has superficial flaking and fine, superficial lines are evident and broken capillaries are common.
- *Mature skin* – the change in the appearance of women's skin during ageing is closely related to the altered production of the hormones oestrogen, progesterone and androgen at the menopause.

Dark skin

On first inspection dark skins usually appear shiny, so it is often presumed that they are greasy, but this is not always the case. Black skins do have more sweat and sebaceous glands and lack the vellus hair that is found on Caucasian and some Asian skins. As black skin has a thicker epidermis, the skin desquamates more than white skin and this may make the skin appear grey. **Erythema** on black skin appears as purple patches. African and Asian skin contains more melanin than Caucasian skin and absorbs almost all the different rays of light, from red right up to ultraviolet. Because of this absorption pattern, it reflects almost no colour so we see it as black or very dark brown. Melanin is a powerful antioxidant, which is why darker skins wrinkle less. Some Asians are very pale with a yellowish undertone due to an inherent tendency to extract beta-carotene from the blood stream and deposit it in the skin. Beta-carotene is also an extremely powerful antioxidant that can scavenge **free radicals** very effectively. The Asian diet is rich in antioxidants (all fruits and vegetables) which act to protect the collagen and elastin in the skin. It is a common misconception that darker, and especially black, skins are tougher than white. In fact, their skin reacts more than Caucasian skin and problems may leave permanent marks and **keloids**. African epidermis is also very sensitive to solar damage even though the deeper layers are better protected, which is another reason why wrinkles are less likely to occur. Although they experience less UV-A damage to the dermis, Africans still suffer from UV-B damage.

Nothing can halt the natural ageing process of any skin type. Collagen will break down over the years and we are all exposed to UV light. However, if the skin is cared for through cleansing, toning, moisturising, eating a good diet rich in fruit and vegetables, using sun blocks, and avoiding toxins like smoking and alcohol, the natural ageing process can be delayed.

ENVIRONMENTAL AND LIFESTYLE FACTORS AFFECTING THE CONDITION OF THE SKIN

Adverse weather conditions

The weather can do untold damage to the skin. Ultraviolet damage is the main culprit, as already discussed at length in this chapter, but the wind and rain and other weather conditions can be just as harmful. Always protect your skin whenever you leave the house. Make sure your moisturiser and/or foundation has a built in sunscreen.

Central heating

Central heating can dry out skin – moisturise the skin daily or use a fine mist spray throughout the day to re-hydrate.

Smoking

Smoking can not only dry out skin, but the continuous action of drawing on the cigarette, can cause vertical lines from the upper lip to the nose. These lines are a sure sign that you are a smoker and are very ageing on a young person.

Drinking alcohol

Drinking any amount of alcohol makes you dehydrated and the skin is the organ that suffers, showing signs of excessive dryness and premature ageing.

Not drinking enough water

The amount of water needed every day depends largely on age, weight, sex and occupation, but an average rule of thumb is between 1 and 2 litres daily. If insufficient water is drunk, the body becomes dehydrated, and this is reflected in poor skin condition.

Weight

An increase in body weight brought about by puberty, pregnancy or just putting on too much weight, may result in stretch marks. Stretch marks can be identified as streaks of thin skin, which are a different colour from the surrounding skin: on a white skin they appear as thin reddish streaks, while on a black skin they appear slightly lighter than the surrounding skin. Whatever the skin colour, the lost elasticity cannot be restored.

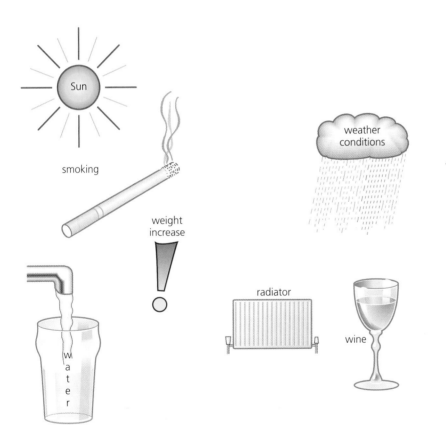

Factors that can contribute to the condition of the skin

Assessment of knowledge and understanding

Knowledge review

1 Which facial muscle, when contracted, gives a frowning expression?

2 Which facial muscle draws the corners of the mouth outwards, giving a smiling expression?

3 Name the skin's three distinct layers.

4 What is the function of the sebaceous glands?

5 State five contra indications to a make-up/facial treatment.

6 What is impetigo?

7 What are the four most common types of sun damage to the skin?

8 What are the symptoms of actinic keratosis?

9 There are many ways you can help prevent sun-damaged skin – list four methods.

10 What is the general treatment for sunburn?

11 What is cryosurgery?

12 What is the best way to reduce the risk of non-melanoma skin cancer?

13 Where do basal-cell carcinomas usually develop?

14 Where do squamous-cell carcinoma usually develop?

15 What is a mole?

16 What does a normal mole look like?

17 What are melanoma warning signs?

18 There are many risk factors for sun-damaged skin, non-melanoma and melanoma skin cancers – list four.

19 Describe a combination skin type.

20 Why does black skin tend to wrinkle less?

chapter 4

Tools of the trade

Brushes, equipment and your make-up kit can be expensive, but you do not need to spend a fortune. Buying the *right* brush, piece of equipment or an item of make-up, however, is more important than the price because the right tool can save you valuable time. Having a collection of different-sized brushes, all with their own specific uses, will allow you to apply and blend colours quickly and easily. For example, using the right sponge will help foundation to go on more easily. It is always tempting to buy cheap products and equipment, but cheaper items may not do the job as well, or may need to be replaced frequently, costing more in the long run. This chapter will advise on the tools of the trade, how to use them, and the pitfalls to watch out for on your shopping trips. Knowledge of the tools of the trade also incorporates knowing about cosmetic and make-up ingredients.

Learning objectives

In this chapter you will learn about:

- **equipment – basic trolley equipment for make-up application**
- **specialist equipment for theatrical make-up**
- **brushes for cosmetic and face painting use**
- **cleansing, toning and moisturising products**
- **concealers, foundations and powders**
- **eye, cheek and lip products**
- **cosmetic ingredients**

TIP

Price doesn't always reflect quality. The most expensive piece of equipment or brush isn't necessarily the best. Shop around.

EQUIPMENT

Basic trolley equipment for a make-up application

The following is a list of the basic items you will need for any make-up application:

- *Brushes* – a full set of quality make-up brushes.
- *Cape, gown or towels* – to protect the model's clothing.
- *Cotton buds.* Round ended ones are excellent for removing make-up. You can also get buds with pointed ends, which are excellent for either applying or removing eye make-up. They allow you to get into the corner of the eye easily, and are more comfortable for the model.
- *Cotton wool* – essential for cleansing – use it dampened.
- *Cotton wool pads* – these have numerous uses, and are especially useful as disposable pads for applying face powder.
- *Disposable brushes* – ideal when making-up many models at once.
- *Eyelash curlers* – used for 'opening up' the eye before mascara is applied. There are two varieties: one curls the whole lash and has handles shaped like scissor handles; the other type are shaped like nail clippers and are good for curling small sections of the eyelash that are difficult to reach. It is worth investing in both types.
- *Hand mirror* – for the model to view the finished result.
- *Headband* – to protect the model's hair.
- *Palette* – for decanting and mixing colours.
- *Sharpener* – an indispensable piece of equipment. Buy one with stainless steel blades and with two different sized sharpening chambers. You will be using this frequently, as every time you use a lip or eye pencil, it must be sharpened before being used on the next model to comply with health and safety regulations.
- *Sponges*
  – natural sponge – for applying cake foundation with water to give a lightweight finish
  – soft sponge – for liquid foundations
  – latex sponge – ideal for applying crème make-up
  – hydra sponge – durable synthetic sponges suitable for most foundations. These sponges are usually 'wedge' shaped for ease of use, and are easily washed.
- *Tissues* – they have numerous uses, such as blotting lipstick.
- *Towels*
- *Tweezers* – these come in many different sizes. You will need angled tweezers for shaping eyebrows.

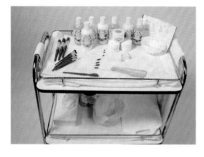

General equipment

Specialist equipment and products for theatrical make-up

In addition to the items listed above, you will also need:

- *Blood* – stage blood can be bought in many different colours and thicknesses to give different effects. Arterial blood is usually a good red, whereas venous blood should be darker. There is also **coagulated** blood, which is perfect for simulating congealed cuts and gashes.
- *Crepe hair* – usually comes in 30 cm tightly woven braids and is used to create beards, moustaches, sideburns and special effects.
- *Hair white* – a water-based liquid for greying hair of all types.
- *Latex* (liquid) – liquid adhesive used to apply crepe hair and prosthetics or to create 'unusual' skin textures.
- *Latex* (tinted) – light flesh and dark flesh shades used for special effects, especially ageing.
- *Spirit gum* – an amber coloured, alcohol/resin liquid adhesive for applying crepe hair, moustaches and beards, wigs, fake noses and bald caps.
- *Spirit gum remover* – a specially developed solvent for the removal of spirit gum.
- *Sponges*
  – stipple sponge – open weave sponge for creating a 'five o'clock shadow' beard, old age spots, bruises and other **stippling** effects.
  – hard sponge – for applying cake foundation with water.
- *Waxes and putty* – products for smoothing the edges on prosthetic pieces, building up facial areas and blocking out eyebrows.

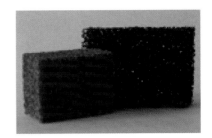

Stippling sponge

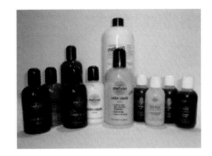

Special effects products from Mehron

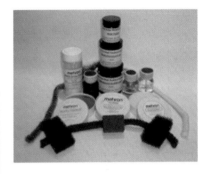

Special effects products from Mehron

HEALTH AND SAFETY

Make-up sponges should be disposed of after use, or washed in warm water and detergent, then placed in a disinfectant solution and rinsed. Allow them to dry, then place them in an ultraviolet cabinet, with each side being exposed for at least 20 minutes.

BRUSHES

To create a particular effect, the right brush must be selected. The brushes used for face painting, for example, are very different to the brushes you would use for a fashion make-up.

- *Face powder brush* – this is the largest brush as it is designed to cover the largest area. It is not restricted to defining shape, its primary purpose being to apply loose face powder to set the foundation.
- *Blusher brush* – used to apply blusher to the cheekbones. It looks similar to the powder brush, but is slightly smaller in order to work more specifically on the cheekbone area.
- *Contour brush* – a smaller brush again than the powder or blusher brush, used to apply contour powder under the cheekbones, and to shade and highlight the face.

- *Foundation applicator brush* – a large brush used specifically to apply liquid foundation. Many make-up artists find using a brush quicker and easier than using sponges. This brush can also be used to apply cream blushers or cream shaders and bronzers.

- *Fan duster* – a feather-fine duster used to gently remove excess setting powder. It can also help to soften the edges of make-up.

- *Eyebrow brush* – a stiff brush to comb into place and shape the eyebrows. Also used in theatrical make-up to apply colour to hair or wigs – white, for example, for ageing.

- *Eyeliner brush* – a very small brush to line the eyes with liquid or cream make-up.

- *Angled brushes* – these come in small, medium and large sizes. They allow angled application of eye shadow, eyeliner and eyebrows.

- *Eye shadow brush* – this should not be too small. Sable brushes are used for product application. These are used for applying eye shadow to the main eye lid area – if the brush is too small, it will take too long to apply the colour.

- *Eye shadow blending brush* – a brush with softer hair that blends powders together without removing the product.

- *Tapered point brush* – for glitter and spot blending of creams and powders.

- *Lip brush* – a firm-tipped, flat lip brush with short thin bristles that gives you good control when applying lipstick and also allows you to build up a deeper shade. Clean thoroughly between models. Disposable lip brushes are available and these are highly recommended.

TIP

Brushes are the most important items in your make-up kit. Always buy the best you can afford. Look after them and they will last a lifetime.

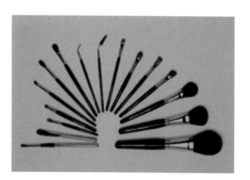

Brushes by Anthony Braden Cosmetics

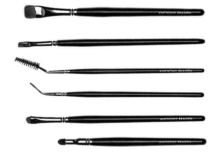

Brushes by Anthony Braden Cosmetics

Face and body painting brushes

There are many brands of brushes designed exclusively for the face painting market. Buying quality brushes from a reputable company is recommended. The Paradise Make-Up AQ® Body and Face painting brushes have custom length handles, luxurious bristles and durable **ferrules** which make them indispensable for the serious artist.

CLEANSING, TONING AND MOISTURISING PRODUCTS

Before any make-up application, the skin must be clean and prepared. Even when you are short of time, it is worth spending adequate time cleansing, toning and moisturising a model's skin prior to any application of make-up. There are numerous products on the market. Some models will bring their own, those to which they know they have no reaction; others allow you to use your own products. It is worth considering buying a hypoallergenic range that will suit most skin types. There are ranges of medical products that not only protect the skin from sun and environmental damage by adding sunscreens, but which also have **antioxidants** added to their products for increased protection. The daily use of a product containing antioxidants protects the skin from free radicals. Free radicals are one of the major causes of ageing, but antioxidants remove them from the skin. The sun, stress, smoking and pollution all generate free radicals. One such product is Skin Ceuticals, which has a medically proven formula and is highly recommended.

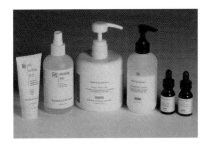

Skin Ceuticals – medically proven products

General cleansing, toning and moisturising products include:

- cleansers
- toners
- moisturisers
- exfoliants
- masks
- massage products
- specialist skin preparations.

CONCEALERS, FOUNDATIONS AND POWDERS

Concealers

Where extra skin coverage is required, it is necessary to apply a special concealer – a cosmetic designed to provide maximum skin coverage. Concealers are usually applied to the skin before foundation.

Foundations

There are many types of foundations, all with different uses and benefits. A kit can only contain so much make-up and in principle, six colours are all that should be needed:

- Fair, medium and dark for white skins.
- Fair, medium and dark for black skins.

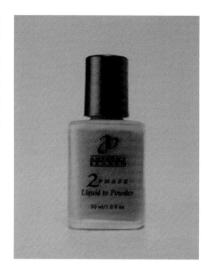

Liquid to powder foundation

Thus, mixing foundations can cater for all skin tones. However, skin tones do vary in the amount of yellow, red and blue they contain, but, with experience, a make-up artist will soon learn which colours to mix to acquire the correct colour.

- *Tinted foundations* – often called tinted moisturisers as they offer a *very* light coverage. They are only used on very clear skin or to enhance a tan. They are often used on young skin, but can also be used as a male foundation – when very little is needed.

- *Liquid foundations* – these are light foundations for everyday use or for a natural look on young or clear skin, often for beauty work. They are applied using a damp sponge or foundation brush onto clean skin. They are usually water based, but can be oil based.

- *Cream foundations* – these provide a thicker coverage, although care must be taken on greasy skins. Often used for older skin or for greater coverage on younger skin. Some cream foundations are designed for everyday use and others, with more pigment, for TV and stage work. Some include powder, although when working under lights, loose powder will often still be needed to set the make-up.

- *Grease foundations* – these are designed for stage work. The advantage of grease make-up is that it provides a good base when a lot of shading is required. It is useful, therefore, for character make-up, but it does require a great deal of powdering.

- *Panstick foundations* – used for heavy coverage as in theatre work. These greasepaints come in palette form or as sticks and have a greater density of pigment. Being greasy, they need powder to set them.

- *Camouflage foundations* – these foundations have a very high pigment content to give greater coverage of the skin. It is designed to disguise skin imperfections such as burns or scars, but is extremely useful for covering unwanted freckles or liver spots caused by ageing. Also used to cover tattoos (see Chapter 12 Camouflage Make-up).

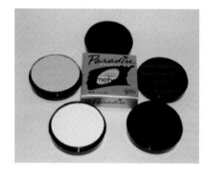

Paradise Aqua colours

- *Pancake foundations* – used for body make-up and where a 'flat' look is required, as on bald heads. Pancake is normally too flat and dry for the face. It does not rub off on clothing, which makes it ideal for use on the body. It is also used for fantasy face painting. Pancakes are water-based foundations, applied using a wet sponge. They dry quickly to a matt finish and when dry can be buffed with a cloth to give a natural looking sheen. Pancake is available in all colours as well as all skin tones.

- *Aqua colours* – these are water-based and come in many lovely colours. They are used for face and body painting and fantasy make-up.

For beauty work, aim for a foundation as near to the natural skin tone as possible. For TV, film and theatre work, anything from one to three shades darker may be required.

Powders

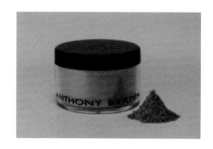

Loose powder

Powder is used for setting make-up. It comes either in a compact, which is good for personal use, or as loose powder, which is better for professional use. Powder comes in a variety of colours but translucent, colourless fine powder is the most versatile and is the most commonly used for professional work. It is helpful if the powder blends with the colour of the foundation; obviously as light, translucent powder has no colour it will not affect the colour of the foundation. This powder can be used on any skin tone, making it very versatile. Powder is used to stop shine and set foundation so that creases do not appear.

EYE, CHEEK AND LIP PRODUCTS

Products for eyes

Eye shadow adds colour and definition to the eye area. There are many varieties of matt and iridescent eye shadows, such as pearlised, metallic and pastel. They are available in cream, crayon or powder form. Eye shadows are composed of either oil and water **emulsions** or waxes containing **inorganic pigments** to give colour. Eye products include:

- *Cream eyes shadows* that contain wax and oil.
- *Crayon eye shadows* – these are composed of wax and oil and are similar in appearance and application to an eye pencil.
- *Powder eye shadows* – these have a talc base, mixed with oils to facilitate application. Lighter shades are produced by the addition of **titanium dioxide** – avoid these on a dark skin as they contrast too harshly with the natural skin colour, resulting in a grey appearance.
- *Pearlised eye shadows* are created by the addition of bismuth oxychloride or mica.
- *Metallic eye shadows* are created by the addition of fine particles of gold leaf, aluminium or bronze.
- *Liquid eyeliner* – defines and emphasises the eye area. Liquid eyeliner is a gum solution in which the pigment is suspended.
- *Powder eyeliner* – this has a powder base with the addition of a mineral oil.
- *Eye pencils* are made of wax and oil, and contain different pigments, which give them colour.
- *Mascara* enhances the natural eyelashes, making them appear longer, darker and thicker. It is available in liquid, cream and block-cake forms. All are composed of waxes or oil and water emulsions, and contain pigments, which give them colour. Liquid mascara can contain short textile filaments, which adhere to the lashes, having a thickening, lengthening effect. Liquid mascara is a mixture of gum in water or alcohol. Water-resistant mascara contains resin instead of gum, so that it will not run or smudge. Cream mascara is an emulsion of oil and water, with the pigment suspended in it. Block mascara is a mixture of mineral oil, **lanolin** and waxes which are melted together to form a block on setting. It must be dampened with water before application.

HEALTH AND SAFETY ✚

If the model has hypersensitive eyes or skin, use hypoallergenic cosmetics that contain no known sensitisers.

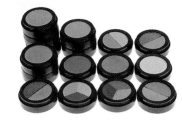

Eye shadow collection by Anthony Braden Cosmetics

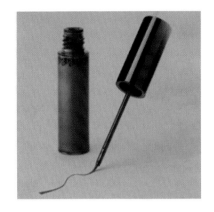

Liquid eyeliner by Anthony Braden Cosmetics

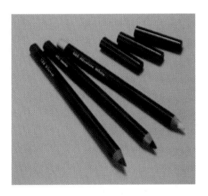

Eye pencils by Anthony Braden Cosmetics

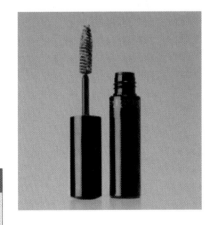

Mascara – white thickening by Anthony Braden Cosmetics

Cheeks

There are two main varieties of products to use on the cheeks: cream blushers and powder blushers. Cream blushers can be used for a 'dewy' look, whereas powdered blushers can be used for a 'matt look'.

Bronzers and shaders

There are literally hundreds of varieties and colours to suit lots of different looks. As with blushers they are available in cream and powder form.

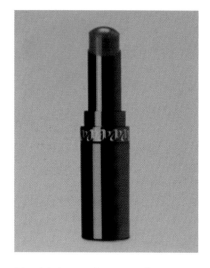

Loose Bronzer by Anthony Braden Cosmetics

Lips

The three main products for the lips are lipsticks, lip glosses and lip liner pencils. Lipsticks contain a blend of oils and waxes, which give them firmness, and **silicone**, essential for easy application. It also contains pigment to add colour, and an **emollient** moisturiser to keep the lips soft and supple. Some lipsticks contain perfume. In addition, they may also include vitamins to condition the lips or sunscreens to protect the lips from UV rays. Lipsticks come in many varieties:

- *cream* – leaves a shiny finish, but needs to be replenished regularly
- *matt* – leaves a dull finish, but is longer lasting
- *frosted* – gives good durability as it is very dry
- *translucent* – colourless lipsticks, not necessarily glossy

Lipstick by Anthony Braden Cosmetics

Lip gloss provides a moist, shiny look to the lips. It may be worn alone, or applied on top of a lipstick. Its effect is short lived. Lip gloss is made of mineral oils, with pigment suspended in the oil. Vaseline can also be used as a lip gloss.

Lip liner pencils may be used to define the lips, creating a symmetrical outline.

HEALTH AND SAFETY ✚
Always sharpen lip liners and eyeliners before their use on a new model, to provide a clean, uncontaminated surface.

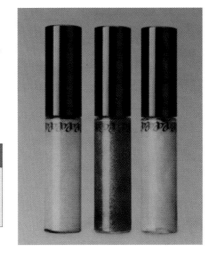

Lip glosses by Anthony Braden Cosmetics

Lip liners by Anthony Braden Cosmetics

COSMETIC INGREDIENTS

Models and clients in beauty salons, while you are applying make-up, will often ask you 'What's in it?' It would be unprofessional to have *no idea* what a product contains. At the same time, it would be almost impossible to know every ingredient used in make-up and cosmetics, but it is recommended that you are aware of the most common ones. You should also be aware of the ingredients that may cause adverse reactions – the two most common are **preservatives** and perfumes. The adverse reaction suffered can come from an **irritant**, from an **allergen** or from a combination of both. Products that contain extracts from animals would be unsuitable for use on many vegetarians. Here are a few examples of ingredients used in cosmetics:

- *Aorta extract* – taken from the aorta, the main artery in animals which transports blood away from the heart. Extracts are used in anti-ageing skin creams.
- *Gelatine* – extracted from collagen, which comes from the bones, skin and white connective tissues of mammals.
- *Lanolin* – a yellowish, viscous wax obtained by refining the wool grease secreted by the sebaceous glands of sheep. Wool grease provides the sheep's fleece with a protective coating. In much the same way, lanolin protects human skin from severe conditions including the weather and central heating. Lanolin moisturises by penetrating the stratum corneum, down to the stratum granulosum (see Chapter 3). Here it holds the moisture (like a reservoir) which can be released to the skin's dry outer layer when necessary. Thus it hydrates the skin, keeping it smooth and closing the cracks that occur in dry skin. This reduces the possibility of invasion by bacteria or viruses.
- *Tallow* (adeps bovis) – obtained from the fatty tissue of cattle and sheep for manufacturing soap. It is also used in shaving cream, shampoo and lipstick production.
- *Thymus extract* – taken from the thymus gland of animals for use in skin creams.

● *Titanium dioxide* – used chiefly in colour cosmetics, and when applied sits on the skin's surface and disperses UV light. It comes in differing particle sizes, generally referred to as 'micro' or 'ultra'. The larger the particles, the more whiteness is left on the skin.

STUDENT ACTIVITY

4.1 Research project

Conduct your own research into the many other ingredients that are contained in cosmetic products.

Assessment of knowledge and understanding

Knowledge review

1 Give three examples of sponges used in make-up and their uses.

2 What does a fan duster brush do?

3 When would you use an angled brush?

4 When would you use a tapered point brush?

5 What is a tinted foundation?

6 What is the difference between a standard make-up and a camouflage make-up?

7 What are aqua colours used for?

8 What is spirit gum?

9 When would you use a stipple sponge?

10 What colour is translucent powder?

11 What would you use to block out eyebrows?

12 Why are disposable mascara brushes recommended?

13 Why should cosmetics containing titanium dioxide be avoided on dark skins?

14 Where is lanolin obtained?

15 What are the two most common ingredients that may cause adverse reactions?

16 What is the purpose of sharpening lip and eye liner pencils before each model?

17 What are lip glosses made from?

18 What would be a good lipstick to recommend to a model with very dry lips?

chapter 5

Before you begin

Before you begin to think about applying make-up, there is preparation work to be done. Preparation includes a visual assessment of the model, observing the facial shape and other characteristics of the face. Preparation also includes either a verbal assessment with the model and the completion of a consultation sheet to ascertain the make-up requirements, or, sometimes, a meeting with a director and make-up designer to ascertain what looks or characters are needed for a certain job. In addition to this research and design stage, preparation also involves cleansing and preparing the skin for make-up.

Learning objectives

In this chapter you will learn about:

- **identifying facial shapes, eyebrow shapes, eye shapes and sizes, lip shapes and sizes**

- **the consultation and consultation sheet**

- **make-up design**

- **research, worksheets and storyboards**

- **preparing the skin for make-up**

HOW TO IDENTIFY FACIAL SHAPES

Your model's features are a major consideration and must be identified before colours and looks can be chosen. There are five basic face shapes, but individuals are often a mixture of these. It is said that an oval face is the perfect shape, but few of us are blessed with a perfect oval face. To analyse a facial shape and to allow you to get an overall picture of the model's features, pull the hair back from the model's forehead and tie it back with a hair band, before examining the bone structure. Look at the cheekbones, the shape of the jaw line, the forehead, the fullness of the cheeks, and pick out the key features. Once you are aware of the true shape of the face, it is much easier to apply blusher, highlighter and contouring products to enhance or hide prominent features.

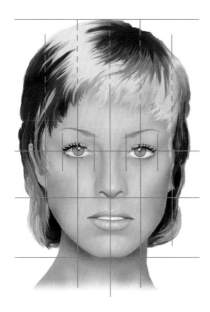

Different facial proportions

It is important to remember that both sides of the face are never the same. We are not 'perfect' and that is what gives each of us our individuality. When doing corrective make-up, for instance, shading a nose or jaw line, try to make sure that the person does not feel that they have something wrong with them.

Drawing the face will also help you to understand its proportions. The face can be divided into equal portions. It can be seen that the eyes are, in fact, halfway between the top of the head and the chin, and the nose halfway between the eyes and the chin. The ears are bigger than is generally thought and are drawn between the eyes and the tip of the nose. The width of the face can also be divided into five sections, each being the width of an eye. Once this 'perfect' face has been understood it can be seen more clearly how individual faces differ.

The five basic face shapes are oval, heart-shaped, round, long and square.

Oval face

The oval face shape has high, sculpted cheekbones with a softly curved jaw line that finishes in a delicate chin. The length of the forehead balances the lower part of the face and the features look regular and neat.

Heart-shaped face

This face is marked by being broad at the top and narrow at the bottom. It can appear long too and the chin pointed and prominent. The cheekbones may be high, but often do not show because of the width of the face.

Round face

Here the forehead, cheeks and chin practically form a circle, which can make features look flat. The cheeks are often plump and full, obscuring the cheekbones.

Long face

This shape can have either a long forehead or a long chin; the features may look drawn and rather raw-boned, creating a tired effect. The cheekbones lack lift because of the length of the face.

Square face

This shape is easily identified by its solid bone structure and square jaw line. The forehead is wide and angled, while the cheekbones tend to be flat and unnoticeable. The cheeks often look plump.

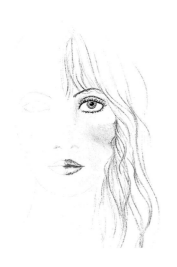

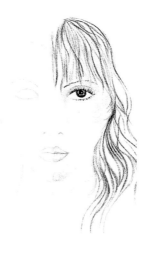

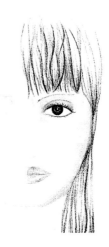

Oval face   Heart face   Round face

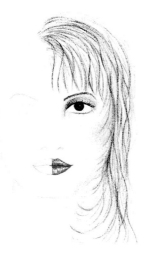

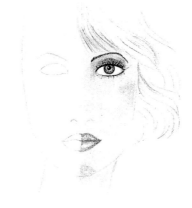

Square face   Long face

A 'combination' of face shapes gives rise to other shapes.

Triangular-shaped face

This shape is similar to the heart shape but has harder features. It is wide at the top and gets thinner as it reaches an almost pointed chin.

Oblong face shape

This is a combination of the square and long face shapes, tending to be flat and unnoticeable and lacking lift.

STUDENT ACTIVITY

5.2   Draw an oblong face and a triangular face shape, in the same format as the basic 5 face shapes.

Eyebrows

Shaping and tinting eyebrows and tinting and perming eyelashes are covered in some detail in the next chapter 'Enhancing the appearance of eyebrows and lashes'. This section will cover the basic eyebrow shapes and discuss which are best fitted to different face shapes. There are five basic eyebrow shapes, with many variations on each one.

The basic eyebrow shapes are as follows:

- *Round* – this shape softens the face, literally adding roundness and helping to tone down sharp features, such as a pointed chin.
- *Angled* – the high, sharp peak draws onlookers' eyes upward, giving a youthful appearance. The peak creates a strong brow that works well with other strong features such as a square jaw. It can also help to make a round or square face appear slimmer. Take care not to angle the brows too sharply or highly as they can look horribly false!
- *Soft angled* – similar to the above, but with a softer and more subtle peak, giving the face a more feminine look. Works well with strong lower face features.
- *Curved* – this is a flattering shape and works especially well on a square or oval face.
- *Flat* – perfect for those with long faces. The horizontal lines of this brow make the face appear shorter and more oval.

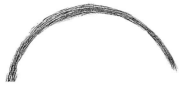

Rounded eyebrow

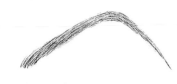

Angled eyebrow

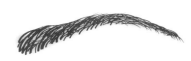

Soft-angled eyebrow

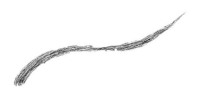

Curved eyebrow

Flat eyebrow

IDENTIFYING EYE SHAPES AND SIZES

Before deciding on any make-up look, you should identify the main features of the eyes.

- *Dark circles under the eyes* – many models, especially Asian models, will have dark circles beneath their eyes. This will be a major factor in the completed make-up look and time will be needed to minimise the darkness with a corrective neutraliser.
- *Wide set eyes* – often people with wide set eyes have a large or wide bridge of the nose. Oriental people generally have wide set eyes.
- *Close set eyes* – people with a thick bridge of the nose often have close set eyes.
- *Round eyes* – round eyes need lengthening or elongating to make them appear longer.

Eyes with dark circles

Wide set eyes

Close set eyes

Round eyes

Prominent eyes

Overhanging lids

Deep set eyes

Downward slanting eyes

Small eyes

Narrow eyes

Oriental eyes

- *Prominent eyes* – or eyes that appear bulging are often caused by **hypothyroidism**, and can be effectively reduced by applying highlighter in other areas to distract attention from the prominent eyes.
- *Overhanging lids* – often seen in older people where gravity is taking its toll.
- *Deep set eyes* – appear deeply set into the skull, often appearing dark and small.
- *Downward slanting eyes* – the eyes dip at the outer corners, often making models look older than they really are.
- *Small eyes* – may be in proportion to the rest of the face, but if not can be 'enlarged' through the right choice of colours and definition.
- *Narrow eyes* – can be opened up through a good choice of make-up colours, eyelash curlers and mascara.
- *Oriental eyes* – often wide set but the main feature is lack of eye lid. Clever make-up techniques can give the illusion of larger eye lids.

IDENTIFYING LIP SHAPES AND SIZES

Very few people have perfect lips, they are often uneven, too small, too large or have an uneven colour. Lips play an extremely important part in any make-up and you will need to be able to make adjustments with your lip colours to hide any imperfections. The ways to achieve these changes will be found in Chapter 7, 'Make-up basics', but here are some of the lip shapes you may encounter.

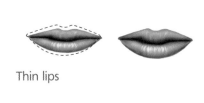

Thin lips

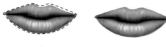

Uneven lips

Full lips

Uneven colour lips

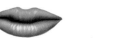

Downward lips

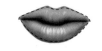

Mature lips

- thin lips
- uneven lips
- full lips
- uneven colour
- downward lips
- mature lips

THE MAKE-UP CONSULTATION

A careful consultation and completed consultation sheet is required before you start to apply any make-up. Never attempt a make-up application with no prior knowledge of what products and colours you are going to apply, and these can only be chosen *after* face, eyebrow, eye and lip shapes and skin type and colours, tones and undertones, have been ascertained. The time it takes to complete a consultation is time very well spent to ensure the model's requirements are met. Imagine completing a make-up look only to find out it did *not* suit the model's requirements. Would you have the time needed to start again? Probably not – a further appointment may have to be made, and you would feel uncomfortable charging for the initial appointment, as you had not done what was required. Adequate time spent on the consultation process, will portray a more professional approach and will instil confidence for the model.

You need to know from the outset the reason the make-up is required. Clients have many reasons for seeking a professional make-up:

- for a complete change of look
- ideas and advice for clients wearing make-up for the first time
- remedial make-up to cover disfigurements or birthmarks (see Chapter 12)
- special occasions:
  - a day out at the races, a graduation party, lunch date, school reunion, shopping day
  - an evening trip to the theatre, dinner party, lecture, concert or just to the pub
  - a wedding – whether as the bride, bride's mother, bridesmaid or guest
  - a christening – mother of the baby, godmother, guest

You also need to know from the outset if the client wants you to do her make-up for a special occasion, or if she in fact wants to make an appointment for a make-up lesson, where the client will apply her own make-up under your instruction. If this is the case, you will need to have booked a longer appointment. (See 'The make-up lesson', Chapter 9.)

If the make-up is for a special occasion, you also need to know if the model requires a trial run. This should be strongly recommended and a special price is usually given for the two combined appointments. In fact, most make-up artists or salons will not do a special occasion make-up without a trial run.

The ideas you may have for the client's final look may be very different from her own ideas, and you cannot assume a client will like your style of make-up choice for her. Therefore, a sensitive approach is essential. Recommend new colours and products by all means, but always be aware of your model's age and any cultural aspects which should be considered. You can start the consultation process as soon as you see the model for the first time, by doing a visual assessment.

- Is her foundation a good colour?
- What colours is she wearing on her eyes and lips?
- What shapes are her eyes and lips?
- What colours are her clothes – are they harmonizing and contrasting or clashing with her make-up choices?
- Does her hairstyle suit her?
- Are there dark circles or bags under her eyes?

A more thorough visual assessment can be made when the client's skin has been cleansed and toned.

Always assess the model's features while she is sitting up, as facial features look very different when lying flat. With the model either on a couch with the backrest in the almost upright position, or with the model sitting in a make-up chair, assess or make notes of the following points:

- skin type – including blemishes, lines and wrinkles
- face shape and colour
- shape of the eyebrows
- shape and size of the lips
- general bone structure
- hair style – does she wear a full fringe or have her hair straight back? What is the colour? Is the colour of her hair the same now as it will be on the day of the special occasion?

Having gathered this important basic information, you need to ask some specific questions regarding the make-up and the model's requirements and expectations of you. Suitable questions are:

- What is the occasion for the make-up?
- What colours do you usually wear?
- Are there any colours you really do not like?
- What do you consider your best/worst features?
- Have you decided on the outfit for the occasion?

● Do you intend to change your hair colour before the occasion?

Record all your findings on the client consultation sheet, which should then be kept in a safe and secure place. The client consultation sheet will also contain all the usual personal information you ask of clients – name, address, contact details, etc. Once you have decided what make-up you will be using, this may be recorded using a separate 'blank face make-up worksheet' record card, which will be kept with the client's consultation form. Whether you have two forms – a consultation form and a blank make-up worksheet – or one comprehensive form is entirely up to you. Designing your own paperwork is a good idea as it will allow you to record the information you want in the way you want to.

Always add an 'outcomes' box to the consultation sheet. You will find this very useful, especially if the end result of the trial make-up is not quite right. The model may request a lighter/darker shade of one product – the lipstick

Example of a blank face worksheet

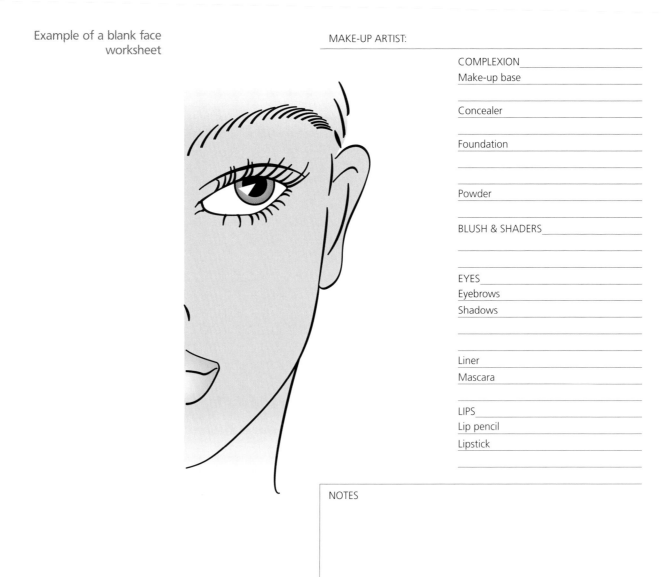

MAKE-UP ARTIST:

COMPLEXION
Make-up base

Concealer

Foundation

Powder

BLUSH & SHADERS

EYES
Eyebrows
Shadows

Liner
Mascara

LIPS
Lip pencil
Lipstick

NOTES

for example – or other small changes for the next application, which will probably be the occasion itself. *Never* memorise colour changes – always write them down. If you are away from the salon on the day of the big occasion, through illness or other unforeseen reasons, another therapist may have to do the make-up and she will need to know *exactly* what to use. A piece of A4 paper with a blank face printed on it is always good for recording your comments and notes. If there is time, you should try out the lighter/darker shade of the adjustment, before the final day. You may also want to include the outfit colours. Either ask to see the outfit or, better still, clip a small piece of fabric sample to the consultation sheet.

STUDENT ACTIVITY

5.3 Designing a consultation and blank face make-up form

Design a make-up record card. Your college may provide one of these for you, however, it may be outdated or may not include all the relevant information you want to include on it. Start with the following general information:

- Name and address
- Contact details
- Date of special occasion (if applicable)
- Skin type/colour/undertone
- Eye and hair colour
- Eyebrow shape and size – is a reshape necessary?
- Lip size and shape

Then allow space for the products you have used in creating the new look and the results

- Foundation   Outcome
- Concealer and/or neutralisers   Outcome
- Eye shadows and liners   Outcome
- Lip colours and lip liners   Outcome
- Mascara colour   Outcome
- Blushers/highlighters   Outcome
- Shaders/bronzers   Outcome

On the day of the final make-up appointment, all you need to have on the trolley are the exact products you will be using. It is too late on the day for anyone's mind to be changed or new products to be tried. This is why the trial make-up appointment is longer than the final application appointment.

MAKE-UP ARTIST PROFILE: VANESSA WAYNE

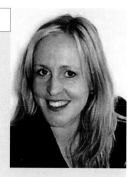

How and when did you start in the business?

I have always had an interest in photography and make-up since school days. In my last year of school, I was a make-up artist for the school play *Wizard of Oz*. My art teacher allowed me to help him develop black and white prints. I was amazed watching images appear from nowhere – it was like magic to me. My dad bought me a camera and I have been taking photographs ever since.

Was there a turning point in your career?

Whilst experimenting with colour photography and make-up, I decided to do a theatrical make-up course. It introduced me to body painting. I have always had a strong interest in photographs that made an impression involving fantasy make-up. Body painting is unique as every body/canvas is different in shape and size, and it continues to change. You can never create the same image twice.

What do you consider to be important qualities for a make-up artist?

Always take care of your model. I believe your model's attitude has a great effect on your work, if your model feels comfortable and good about themselves their feelings will shine through and can affect your work more positively. Personal hygiene is important. Patience and a positive attitude attract clientele.

What is your most memorable/exciting/best paid job?

I worked at the Glastonbury children's festival weekend in 1993. My pay was free entry for family and friends if I worked as a face painter for a few hours. I enjoyed it so much I worked all day. I had a long queue of children and the joy on their faces was a pleasure to see. The children's festival's aim was and still is to raise money to run workshops for children who have 'special needs'.

Have you had any disasters?

I nearly had a big disaster once in a studio. We left the studio for only a minute to touch up the body paint in the next room. On our return we could smell smoke – the backdrop had fallen down on top of a very hot lamp. We did, however, have an extinguisher at hand.

What advice would you give to young people entering the industry?

Go for it. Don't give up too easily and get as much experience as possible. Think positively even when you make mistakes, because you learn from your mistakes. Always have an open mind to learn new things and try new ideas. Always be punctual and reliable even if you are working for free, even the seemingly insignificant jobs can bring unexpected rewards.

In your experience, would you advise those training to become make-up artists to specialise in one area only, or to gain experience, through Continued Professional Development courses (CPD) in many different areas of make-up?

Specialising in one area is good, but there is a natural progression. Have a go at everything – there is always something new to learn. If you can't afford the cost of fees, buy your make-up, paint or prosthetics and practise on a friend or practise on yourself. My first model for body painting was myself. I started on my legs and worked my way up, obviously I could only paint my front half of my body. You can also experiment with casualty. Give yourself black eyes, scars on your arms or legs. Bald cap is a bit tricky. However, if you can afford courses then go on as many as you can.

MAKE-UP DESIGN AND RESEARCH

The earlier description of the consultation is typical of a beauty salon procedure, when the make-up look will be determined by the client with the recommendations and practical skills of the make-up artist or therapist. With other work, such as fashion, editorial, catalogues, pop videos, it may be that the make-up look is determined by the make-up designer and the rest of the team, and merely applied by the make-up artist.

Planning

Make-up artists working in areas other than beauty salons and spas will need to complete considerably more paperwork. The make-up professional should be involved with the planning stages of any production, right from the start, especially for a character that may require not only make-up but prosthetics and/or postiche work as well. It may be that you only have to produce such a character as a one-off, or you may have to recreate it over and over again. Either way, you will have to plan and research the character and work with the director and crew. Two of the most important people, other than the director, that the make-up artist should be involved with are the lighting personnel and the photographers, as they can all be of tremendous help to you and your work.

If the make-up is going to create a character in a play or a film, that character may have to develop over a period of time. In this case, a 'storyboard' has to be produced, so that everyone involved can see the development of the character through all of its stages. This may have been done for you, or you may find that you have to produce a storyboard yourself. On occasion, you may stand in for the regular make-up artist at some point and have to work to their make-up plans and storyboards. You will soon realise why it is so important for make-up artists to attend meetings and put as much information as possible into the plans from the outset. Even if you are the make-up assistant, showing commitment to the production will always go in your favour – should the regular make-up artist be unable to work for any reason, you will undoubtedly be asked to stand in. It cannot be stressed enough how important continuity is, in this situation, and how valuable make-up plans and storyboards are, so keep them clear and make sure you have all the relevant points and notes clearly marked on them. For a one-off character, you may only need a standard consultation and a blank make-up worksheet, but make sure that you still put all the information needed to create the character on the form. When the paperwork is finished with, file it safely for future reference. You will find that storyboards are mainly used in the film industry and are a great way of showing everyone exactly what is needed without too much explanation. They can be found in lots of different forms and formats, from individual boards to boards with multiple sections that resemble comics. Of course nowadays a lot of storyboards are created on computers, making it easy to store, reproduce and send them to anyone who may need such information.

EQUIPMENT AND PRODUCT LIST
Equipment and products for The Road to Oz
Equipment
Selection of sponges and brushes
Products
Yellow Mehron liquid make-up
Yellow Grimas make-up
White cream make-up stick
Silver Mehron metallic powder
Mehron mixing liquid
Grimas gold cream make-up
Red Grimas cream
Black eyeliner
Black eye shadow powder
White translucent powder

Body painting – the Road to Oz

The Road to Oz was a body painting designed for a competition. The first illustration shows the artist's ideas on paper. Even before getting to this stage, there would have been hours of researching into the different characters and aspects of the film *The Wizard of Oz*. This is an excellent interpretation, incorporating several characters and aspects of the film and it deserved the winning prize it achieved at a make-up competition.

The painting was created as follows.

Black eyeliner was used to draw the bricks; the bricks on the face were filled with yellow cream, with white cream used for the lines between the bricks. All were carefully powdered and then a black powder eye shadow and a brush were used to touch up the black lines.

Yellow and gold creams were blended to create the gold lion on the other side of the face. Bronze cream was also used in places. On one side of the body, silver metallic powder was used under the chin and on the body and a dark blue face paint created the nuts and bolts of the tin man's elbows, knees and ankles. The red poppies in the hair were cut out from red card and held in place with a hair clip pushed through a tiny hole in the black centre of the poppy.

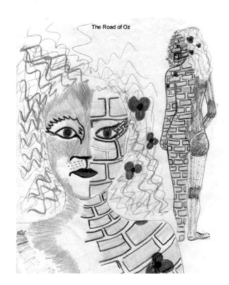

Road to Oz sketch

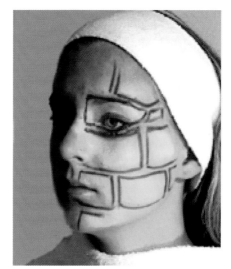

Road to Oz stage 1

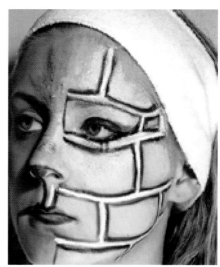

Road to Oz stage 2

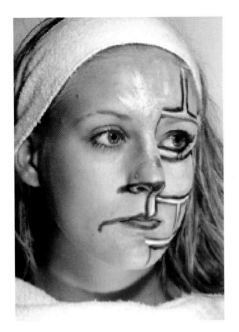

Road to Oz stage 3

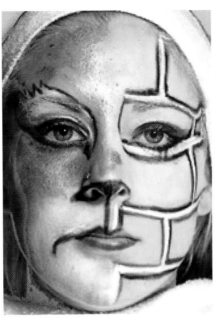

Road to Oz stage 4

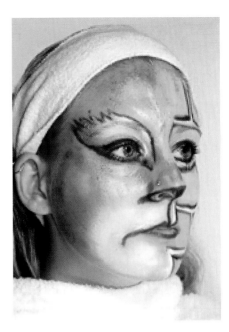

Road to Oz stage 5

Road to Oz final

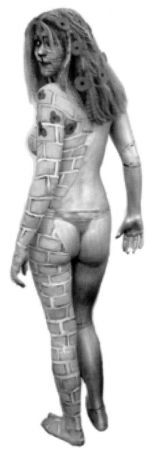

Road to Oz

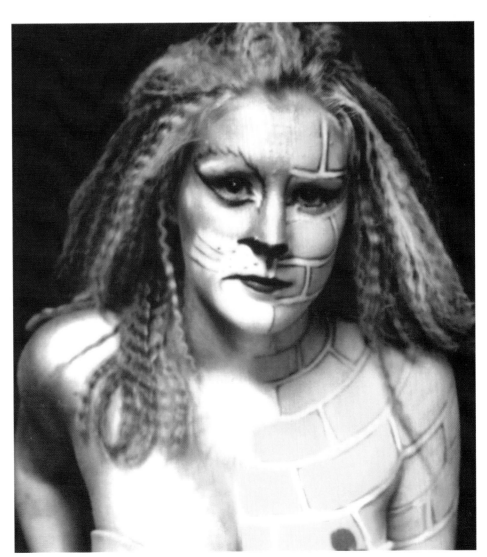

Research

Where do you start researching a character? If it is a historical figure, or anyone who actually lived, then the Internet is the place to start. Key in the character's name and see what turns up. On the Google homepage (www.google.co.uk), you can opt for an image search, which may be especially fruitful. Print off only what looks interesting to your needs. You can also research books in a library and maybe take out a biography or autobiography and read about the character. Pictures are sometimes not always enough – if you can learn more about a character by reading about them and getting a feel for the life they led, it will become easier to re-create their features on a model.

If you are researching a fictional character and need some help with ideas, you can look through websites from film, television, theatre, sci-fi, horror and futuristic sites – you may come across a feature from another character that will set you off towards creating your own new character. Look for colour, shape, design and generally inspirational ideas. Sometimes, however, you can get so loaded with images that you have to create something entirely from your own imagination. It can be very inspirational just sitting somewhere 'people watching'.

PREPARING THE SKIN FOR MAKE-UP – CLEANSING, TONING AND MOISTURISING

If you are working 'on the road', there is only so much kit you can carry around with you, so choose a range of cleansers, toners and moisturisers that will suit the majority of skin types. A hypoallergenic range is always a good choice. However, some models will have their own products for you to use, in fear of being allergic to any new product you may have. If you work in the luxury of a beauty salon, you will have access to all the skin ranges, so choose one that suits your model's skin type. Many models arrive without make-up, so you may only need to use a facial wipe before you begin. Alternatively, you may only have time to do a simple cleanse, tone and moisturise. However, it is strongly emphasised that the more time you spend on preparing the skin for make-up, the better the end result will be. Now there follows a sequence for a basic cleanse, tone and moisturise. In addition, there are further steps for a 'double cleanse', tone and moisturise. The length of time required for these treatments makes them suitable for beauty salons and spas.

1 Having washed your hands, prepare the model by placing a hairband around the hair to expose all the face and neck areas to be cleansed. The model will be lying on a treatment couch, and the make-up artist or therapist will be seated at the model's head.

2 Start by cleansing the eyes, one at a time, with a suitable eye make-up remover, and cotton wool pads. Each eye is cleansed separately. Your non-working hand lifts and supports the eye tissue whilst the working hand applies the eye make-up remover. Always follow the manufacturer's

instructions on the product you have chosen to use. The eye area is cleansed in circular movements, outwards over the upper lid, and then under the lashes towards the nose. Repeat a few times until the cotton wool pads are clean, and all the old eye make-up has been removed. You may need to use a cotton bud under the lashes if old make-up was not removed with first cleansing.

3   Cleanse the lips of old lip colour by applying a cleansing product to the lips and gently massaging the product into the lips with circular movements – usually with a clean finger or a cotton bud. Remove the cleanser with a clean damp cotton pad, from the upper lip first, with firm pressure from right to left and then the bottom lip, from left to right. Continue these moves until there is no trace of old lip colour left.

4   Apply cleanser to the face, according to the manufacturer's instructions, and gently cover the face and neck with the product. You may need to warm the product first in your hands before applying it to the model. Working from the neck upwards, towards the forehead, use long sweeping and light circular movements, gently massaging the product into the skin. Never drag the skin, and avoid sensitive areas around the eyes.

5   Remove the cleanser thoroughly with clean damp cotton pads, again working from the neck upwards and outwards. Concentrate on the areas around the nose, in the lines of the forehead and in the crease of the chin, where old make-up accumulates. Repeat until the damp cotton pads are clean, and all cleanser has been removed from the skin.

If you are doing a basic cleanse, you would now tone the skin – go to Step 13. Continue with the instructions below for the 'double cleanse' treatment.

6   Having removed all the surface dirt and grime with the first cleanse, you are now going to repeat step 4 again, but this time including more massage movements over a longer time period. There are many sequences, all of which are acceptable and achieve the desired outcome of a perfectly clean skin on which to apply make-up products. Apply more cleansing product to the hands, warming it if necessary and apply to the neck and face areas. Stroke up either side of the neck, using your fingertips. At the chin, draw the fingers outwards to the angle of the jaw, and lightly stroke back down the neck to the starting position.

7   Apply small circular movements over the skin of the neck area.

8   Using your hands alternately, stroke the jawbone and chin, really working the cleansing product into this area.

9   Now, from the chin area, using your middle fingers, make circular movements over the chin, up the sides of the nose and over to the temples, still working the cleansing product into the skin. Keep all movements slow but firm, and really concentrate on what you are doing.

10 From the forehead and using your middle and ring fingers, run your fingers down the nose using alternate hands.

11 With the ring fingers, and cleansing one eye at a time, trace a circle around the eye sockets. Begin at the inner corner of the upper brow bone and slide to the outer corner, around and under the eyes, over the bridge of the nose to the starting position. Do this several times and then repeat to the other eye.

12 Still using the middle and ring fingers, apply small circular movements across the forehead – several times.

13 After the skin has been cleansed, it is then toned with the appropriate toning lotion. Following the manufacturer's instructions, tone the skin, removing all traces of the cleansing products. The most usual method of applying toner is on two cotton wool pads, working from the neck up to the forehead. Continue with the toning lotion until the skin is perfectly clean, and there are no traces of product left on the pads.

14 Make a small tear in the centre of a large facial tissue, for the model's nose. Place the tissue over the face and neck and mould it into position to absorb excess moisture from the toning lotion.

15 The choice of moisturiser would depend on the model's treatment. In this case, the cleansing is prior to a make-up application, and so a very small amount of a light moisturiser would be appropriate.

16 Once you start applying the foundation for the make-up, if you find that more moisturiser is needed, it can be applied at this time.

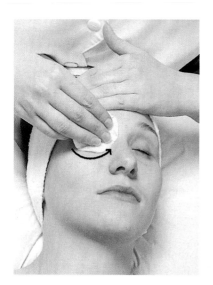

Cleansing the eye area

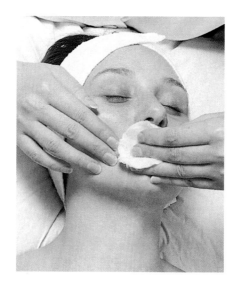

Cleansing the lips

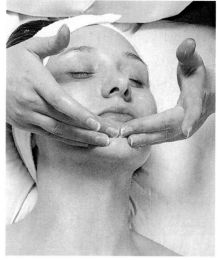

Cleansing the face

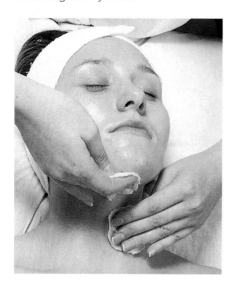

Removing cleanser

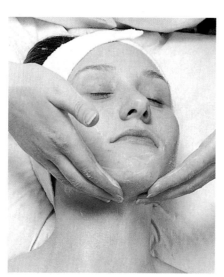

Applying cleanser

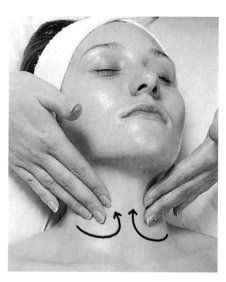

Circular manipulations of the neck

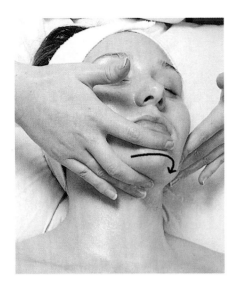

Stroking the jawbone and chin

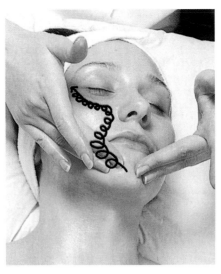

Circular manipulations of the chin, nose and temples

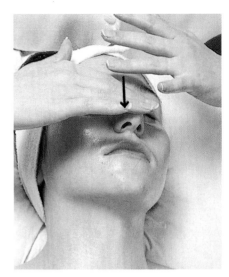

Running movement on the nose

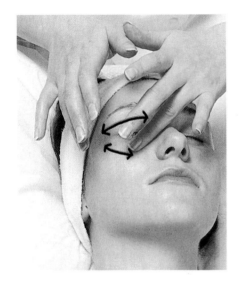

Eye circling

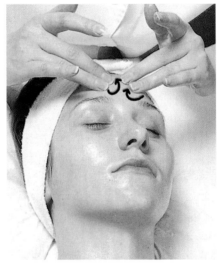

Circling of the forehead

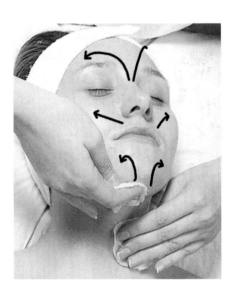

Toning

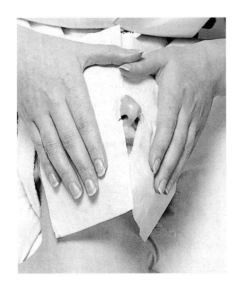

Blotting the skin

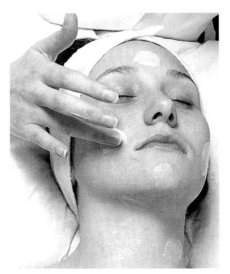

Applying moisturisers

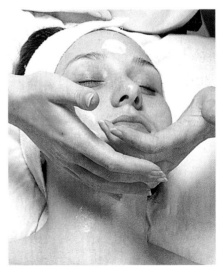

Applying moisturisers

The cleaning process is usually applied with the therapist sitting behind the model. Once this has been completed, the model would sit up on the couch and the therapist would face the model, ready for the application of make-up.

If you removed any of the model's outer clothing for the cleansing process, you may now like the model to replace them. You would not want a good make-up spoiled by a model pulling a jumper over her head. In fact, it is recommended that if a model comes to a salon for a make-up application, you advise them to wear something that does not have to go over the head.

Assessment of knowledge and understanding

Knowledge review

1 How many basic face shapes are there, and what are they?

2 What is commonly described as the 'perfect' face shape?

3 How would you describe a heart shaped face?

4 How many basic eyebrow shapes are there and what are they?

5 Name four different lip shapes.

6 Why is it necessary to complete a client consultation sheet?

7 Give three reasons why a client may book into a beauty salon for a make-up application.

8 Name three types of immediate visual assessment.

9 Why should you always assess the client's features while she is sitting up?

10 What are storyboards?

11 How would you use a blank face make-up form?

12 Why is it important to be involved with the planning of any film or theatrical production right from the start?

chapter 6

Enhancing the appearance of eyebrows and eyelashes

This chapter looks at how to enhance the appearance of the eyebrows and eyelashes, a fundamental part of any make-up application. Eyebrow re-shaping, eyelash and brow tinting, and eyelash perming are popular salon treatments, so it is imperative for beauty therapists to be fully competent with these treatments. However, it is also important for make-up artists to be proficient in this area too. A make-up application for a wedding or special occasion, in fact any make-up, can be spoiled if the eyebrows are undefined or unkempt; in magazine photos every eyebrow hair can be seen and so must be perfectly shaped. This chapter deals with the enhancement of eyebrows and lashes by shaping eyebrows using tweezers, tinting eyebrows and lashes, and perming eyelashes. Chapter 7, 'Make-Up Basics', will cover redefining and shaping brows using make-up, Chapter 10, 'Wigs and Postiche', will show you how to apply false lashes and Chapter 11, 'Theatrical and Media Make-Up', will explain how to block out eyebrows in order to redesign and achieve a specific look.

Learning objectives

In this chapter you will learn about:

- eyebrow shaping
- eyelash and brow tinting
- eyelash perming

SKIN TESTS

A skin test, also known as a patch test or a hypersensitivity test, needs to be carried out before each lash or brow tinting treatment – even if the client has had a treatment with you before. Some clients become allergic with continued use of a product, whilst others produce an allergic reaction

HEALTH AND SAFETY

Skin test – always carry out a skin sensitivity test at least 24 hours prior to an eyelash tint. Eyelash tints can irritate and cause adverse reactions. Always refer to the manufacturer's instructions and COSHH regulations when using chemical products.

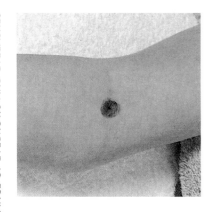

Skin test

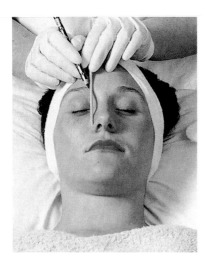

Measuring the eyebrow: the inner eye

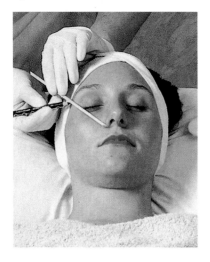

Measuring the eyebrow: the outer eye

immediately upon contact with the product. If you carry out any eyelash or brow tinting treatment *without* doing a skin test, and there is a reaction, you are likely be in default of your insurance cover. Always carry out the patch test 24 hours prior to the treatment and test behind the ear or in the crook of the elbow. Mix the tint according to the manufacturer's instructions and apply to the test area with a small disposable brush, and allow to dry. The tint should be left on the skin for 24 hours before being washed off and the model should watch out for any reactions. If a reaction occurs, the tint should be removed immediately with warm water and a soothing lotion applied to the area.

Two responses to the skin test are possible:

- a negative result which produces no skin reaction – in which case you may proceed with the treatment
- a positive result which produces irritation, swelling and inflammation on the skin – in which case you *cannot* proceed with the treatment.

Contra indications to all eye enhancing treatments include:

- a positive reaction to any product after a skin test
- skin diseases or disorders including conjunctivitis, stye or **blepharitis**
- viral infections – including a severe common cold
- active eczema or psoriasis
- contact lenses – unless removed
- bruising to the eye area
- any inflammation or swelling around the eye.

EYEBROW SHAPING

A make-up artist is likely to use the tweezing method for eyebrow shaping and will usually only have to tidy up stray brows rather than a total eyebrow reshape. Beauty therapists, on the other hand, will often be faced with a total reshape of the eyebrows and may decide to remove the hairs by tweezing, depilatory waxing or **threading** as methods of reshaping. All these methods are temporary measures and the model will have to return approximately every four weeks after the hair has re-grown for further treatment. Some therapists may suggest more permanent ways of hair removal using electrical methods.

In a beauty salon the recommended treatment time for eyebrow shaping is 15 minutes, although if a complete reshape is being undertaken 30 minutes may be needed. Thorough model consultation procedures must be carried out before performing these treatments to ensure you carry out the model's wishes and she has a full understanding of the treatment. Chapter 5 explains model consultations in detail. If the model is considering this treatment before any special occasion make-up, then timing must be a main consideration. As eyebrow shaping may cause erythema, it is recommended the model comes in for the eyebrow shape a day or two before the special occasion, so that all erythema will have gone and the make-up application will have a better final result.

A make-up artist may not have the opportunity to pre-shape the eyebrows before a make-up application. In this case, tweeze only the hairs that are unattractive and need to be removed, and then wipe the brows over with antiseptic lotion. You may want to start work on another aspect of the make-up and return to the eyebrows when any redness has diminished.

Refer to previous chapter to see which eyebrow shapes are best suited to which face shapes.

To balance the eyebrows take an orange stick, or something similar, and draw a vertical line directly from the outside edge of the nostril upwards – this is where the inner edge of the eyebrow should start. Then join up the edge of the nostril to the outer edge of the eye – the continuing diagonal line will show you where the outer edge of the eyebrow should end.

Another way of measuring if the eyebrow is balanced is by drawing a vertical line from its lower inner edge to its outer edge. If this line is a straight horizontal line, the eyebrows are balanced.

- If the line goes up at the outer edge, you will have to draw in some brows at the outer edge to bring the line down again so it is horizontal.
- If the line goes down, you will have to fill in the inner brow to balance the line again.

The illustrations will give you some examples.

Step-by-step eyebrow shaping

1 Wash your hands. Ensure you have everything ready in the work area, sterilised and accessible.

2 Carry out the consultation, discussing model's requirements and checking for contra indications.

3 Remove contact lenses if necessary.

4 With the model lying comfortably on the couch, measure the eyebrows as detailed above.

5 Cleanse the area to be treated and wipe with sanitising lotion.

6 Brush the brows into shape before you begin.

7 Remove eyebrow hairs carefully and effectively, grasping the hair near the surface of the skin with your preferred tweezers, and tweeze in the direction of hair growth to achieve the desired shape.

8 Dispose of the removed hairs hygienically and sanitize tweezers again.

9 Apply a mild antiseptic or soothing substance at the end of the treatment.

10 Show the model the finished results and record details of the treatment on the model's record card.

11 Advise the model to wear no make-up for 12 hours after treatment.

12 Complete the service in the given time.

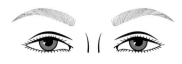
A balanced eyebrow

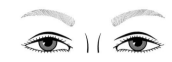
An eyebrow too short at the outside edge

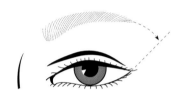
Adjusted eyebrow to make balanced

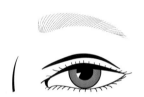
An eyebrow too high on the inside edge

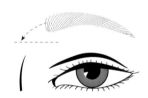
Adjusted eyebrow to make balanced

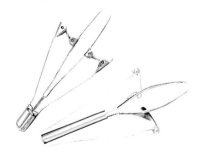
Automatic tweezers

EQUIPMENT AND PRODUCT LIST

Equipment and products for eyebrow shaping

Equipment

Orange stick for measuring

Eyebrow brush

Tweezers (rounded/slanted/pointed)

Damp cotton wool

Antiseptic lotion

After care solution

Disposable gloves

Tissues

Lined container for waste

Hand mirror

Client record card

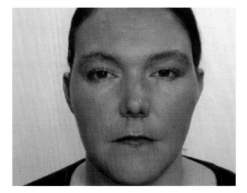

Before reshaping treatment

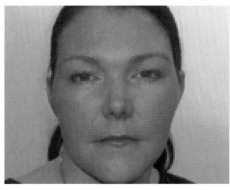

After reshaping treatment

TIP

To remove hairs more easily, you can place warm, damp cotton pads over the eyebrows for a minute or so. This relaxes the hair follicles and softens the eyebrow tissue. If you are shaping your own eyebrows at home, the best time is after a warm bath or shower.

HEALTH AND SAFETY

Blood may be drawn during an eyebrow shape. Apply pressure with a cotton wool pad soaked in sanitising solution before applying soothing lotion. Dispose of waste materials according to Health & Safety regulations and the by-laws of your area.

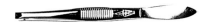

Manual tweezers

HEALTH AND SAFETY

Always use a tint that is manufactured specifically for eyelash and eyebrow tinting and is permitted for use under EU regulations. Always follow the manufacturer's instructions carefully. Not to do so may render your insurance invalid.

HEALTH AND SAFETY

Never leave the model alone when performing an eyelash or eyebrow tint. If the tint goes into the eye, you must be on hand to remove product immediately. If you leave the room and something happens to your model, your insurance company may not compensate.

EYEBROW AND EYELASH TINTING

The hair of the eyelashes and eyebrows protects the eyes from moisture and dust, but the lashes and brows also give definition to the eye and a frame to the face. Many models, especially those with fair lashes and brows, feel that without the use of eye cosmetics their eyes lack this definition. Definition of the brows and lashes can be obtained if a permanent dye is applied to them.

Products for eyelash and eyebrow tinting are available in creams or gels and usually come in the basic colours of blue, black, grey and brown. Colours can be mixed to get the desired result. Blue and black mixed together, for example, will give a darker colour. The choice of colour will be the model's decision, but you can advise on suitability.

Developing times

The developing time for eyelash tinting depends on the natural colour of the hair. Blond and fair hair develops rapidly, that is roughly 5 minutes. Red hair is more resistant and development will take longer, say 10 minutes. Eyebrows take far less time to develop, taking approximately 1 to 3 minutes – so never leave the model alone and check frequently.

Step-by-step eyelash tinting

Check that a patch test has been carried out and that there was a negative result.

1 Ensure that all equipment has been sanitised and is close to hand.

2 Carry out the model consultation and check for contra indications.

3 Remove contact lenses, if necessary.

4 Cleanse the area with a non-oily product – removing all traces of make-up.

5 Apply a barrier cream like Vaseline to the skin, and apply pre-formed shapes under the eyelashes.

6 Mix tint immediately prior to application. With model's eyes open, cover the lower lashes with tint before asking model to close their eyes and apply tint to upper lashes. Make sure you reach the roots of the lashes.

7 If the model complains of discomfort or the eyes begin to water, remove the tint immediately using damp cotton wool pads, and irrigate the eye.

8 Note the time and allow time for the tint to work according to the manufacturer's instructions. The colour should be checked at intervals and the tint reapplied if necessary. As a guide allow 5–10 minutes depending on the colour characteristics of the model. Note processing time on model's record card.

9 Remove tint, one eye at a time, after the required processing time, or when you can see that the tint has taken to the required colour. Place a damp pad of cotton wool over the eye. Hold the eye shield and pad of cotton wool together at the base and swiftly remove, enclosing any excess tint. Remove any remaining tint with slightly damp cotton wool, using a gentle downward and outward motion, and remove excess with a cotton bud. When both eyes have been cleaned, ask the model to carefully open her eyes. Support the eye and work quickly on the lower lashes with damp cotton wool and cotton buds, removing any excess tint.

10 Show your model the results and give after care advice.

11 Record details on the model's record card.

EQUIPMENT AND PRODUCT LIST
Equipment and products for eyelash tinting
Equipment
Protective headband and towel
Couch roll to protect the work area
Small glass bowl for mixing tint
Lined container for waste
Sterile spatula
Orange sticks
Small bowl of clean cool water
Hand mirror
Model record card
Products
Non-oily eye make-up remover
Vaseline or barrier cream
Eyelash and brow tint in various colours (black, brown, blue and grey)
Hydrogen peroxide
Damp cotton wool and tissues
Eye shields made from cotton pads or paper shields

HEALTH AND SAFETY

Never do an eyelash or brow tint when there has been an adverse reaction. Do not use a higher strength than 10-volume or 3% hydrogen peroxide. If you do, skin irritation or minor skin burning may occur.

Step-by-step eyebrow tinting

Eyebrow tinting can be performed after lash tinting and prior to eyebrow shaping. The eyebrows take very quickly, and the treatment can be performed whilst the eyelash tint is developing. This also makes very good use of your time. If you perform an eyebrow tint alone, the treatment time is

15 minutes and is not cost effective. The effects of the treatment will last approximately 4–6 weeks as the hairs grow out. Strong sunlight will make the results fade faster.

You will need the same equipment as for an eyelash tint.

1 Prepare the skin and brows the same way as for treating the lashes. Apply barrier cream around the eyebrows taking care to avoid any hairs you want tinted.

2 Brush the hairs against hair growth, and apply tint with an orange stick or fine brush, working from the outside in.

3 After applying tint to the second eyebrow, immediately check the first to assess development. The developing time for tinting eyebrows is much shorter than for lashes – usually between one and three minutes.

4 When the lashes are dark enough, remove the tint with clean damp cotton wool, removing all traces of tint.

5 Remove all traces of barrier cream.

6 Show the model the finished result and enter details on the model's record card.

After care advice for eyelash and eyebrow tinting

- Model should not touch or rub the areas just treated.
- If redness or irritation occurs, bathe with damp cotton wool.

ENHANCING THE APPEARANCE OF EYELASHES

Some eyelashes need no specific treatment other than the use of eyelash curlers. Eyelash curlers 'open up' the eye area, enhancing the make-up and allowing you to see the colour of the model's eyes. This is an excellent technique for oriental models who tend to have long, very straight eyelashes. However, as prolonged use can lead to a deterioration of the eyelashes, curlers should be used for special occasions only.

EYELASH PERMING

With mechanical methods of eyelash curling leading to a deterioration of the eyelashes, eyelash perming offers a safe alternative. The use of perming solutions, although chemically based, are far less damaging than the regular use of eyelash curlers. Eyelash perming entails permanently curling the lashes, which helps to emphasise the eyes and eliminates the daily use of eyelash curlers and mascara. Eyelash perming gives immediate effects. It promises a curled effect, even when wet, for up to six weeks. Eyelash perming is recommended for:

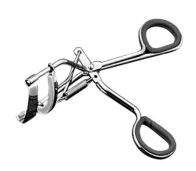

Eyelash curlers

HEALTH AND SAFETY

Repeated use of eyelash curlers can lead to breakage. Only use the technique for special occasions.

TIP

The perming lotion has a slight, but unavoidable odour. Treatment should be carried out in a well-ventilated area.

- Oriental eyes – or any eyes that are downward slanting – the eyes appear lifted when the outer lashes are curled
- models who wear contact lenses or glasses
- for special occasions
- for models who have short, straight and sparse lashes to make them appear longer and denser
- for regular sportswomen
- for holidays
- for models who do not wish to, or cannot, wear mascara.

The treatment is unsuitable for:

- lashes that are fragile
- lashes that are *very* short and sparse
- naturally curly lashes

TIP

Do not tint eyelashes before perming, as the treatment process may lighten the colour of the lashes. Eyelash tinting is very effective following eyelash perming and should be encouraged.

Step-by-step eyelash perming

Ensure that a skin test has been carried out before making a firm appointment for eyelash perming.

1 Thoroughly cleanse the eye and lashes, using a non-oily remover, removing all traces of make-up.

2 Choose suitable sized rods (curlers), depending upon the lashes and the curl required.

3 Apply a small amount of adhesive to the main body of the rod. Check that no lashes are caught underneath. Bend and shape the rod to sit tightly but comfortably in the eye shape, and curl the lashes over the rods.

4 When you are satisfied that the lashes are straight apply perm lotion evenly to the upper lashes, using a disposable brush.

5 Cover the lashes with plastic film or dry lint-free pads. This creates warmth, which aids the perming process.

6 Remove the perm lotion using dry lint-free pads, gently blotting the lashes.

7 Apply fixing lotion with a clean disposable brush (according to the manufacturer's instructions).

8 Cover the lashes with plastic film or dry lint free pads for 10–15 minutes.

9 Gently remove the fixing solution from the lashes, using dry lint free pads, and remove each curler, rolling downwards.

10 Apply moisturising product.

11 Wipe any excess products from lashes with damp clean cotton wool and show the model the finished result.

EQUIPMENT AND PRODUCT LIST

Equipment and products for eyelash perming

Equipment

Towels

Headband

Fixing lotion

Eyelash curlers – different sizes

Eyelash adhesive

Lint free pads + bowl

Orange sticks

Disposable brushes – to apply perm and fixing lotion

Damp cotton wool + bowl

Bottle with long flexible tube

Lined dish for waste materials

Hand mirror

Client record card

Products

Eye make-up remover (non-oily)

Perm solution – especially designed for use in the eye area

HEALTH AND SAFETY

Products vary – always follow the manufacturer's instructions.

HEALTH AND SAFETY

Protective gloves may be worn to reduce the risk of chemical contact with the skin.

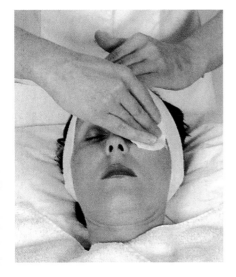

Cleansing the eye area

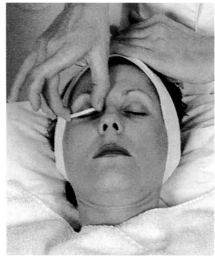

Selecting the correct curler

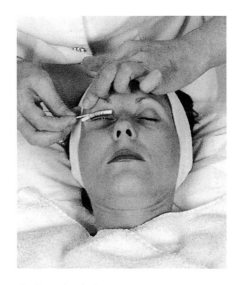

Curling the lashes

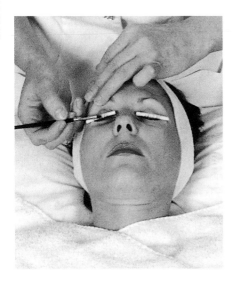

Applying the perm lotion

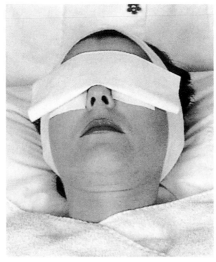

Processing the perm lotion

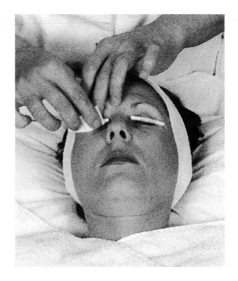

Removing the perm lotion

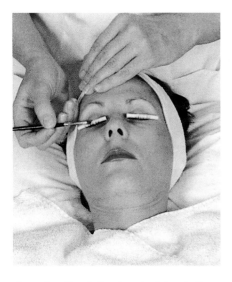

Applying the fixing/neutralising lotion

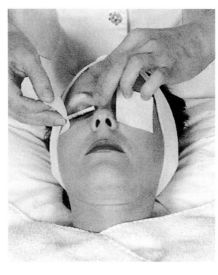

Covering the lashes with lint-free pads

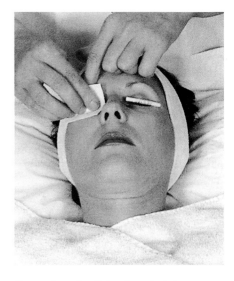

Removing the fixing/neutralising lotion

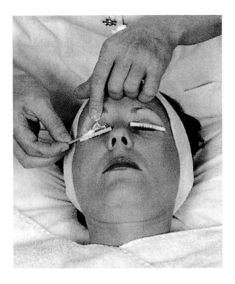

Removing the curler

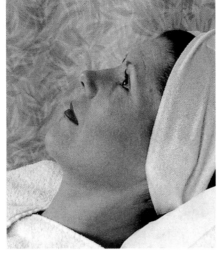

The completed effect

HEALTH AND SAFETY ✚

If the model complains of discomfort during the treatment, the chemical lotion may have entered the eye. Remove perm lotion immediately using clean damp cotton wool pads. Flush eye if necessary with distilled water dispensed directly from the water bottle.

TIP ✔

Always replace the cap tightly after use as perming lotion loses its strength each time it is exposed to the air.

Eyelash perming troubleshooting

- If the treatment resulted in the lashes being too curly, you probably used a rod that was too small. You can re-perm with a larger rod.

- If there appears to be no result, you either used a rod that was too big, there was insufficient processing, and/or incorrect neutralising or you may have left an oil barrier on the lashes. You will have to re-perm.

- If you were left with an uneven curl, you positioned the rod incorrectly, or applied the perming gel unevenly or did not curl the lashes over the rod properly. You will have to re-perm, repositioning the rod.

- If the lashes were buckled or hooked at the ends, then you incorrectly wrapped the lashes around the rod. You could carefully trim off the ends.

TIP ✔

Eyelash perming products should be stored in a cool, dark and safe place.

Assessment of knowledge and understanding

Knowledge review

1 How would you measure for the correct eyebrow shape?

2 What is the recommended time for eyebrow shaping and reshaping?

3 How should the brow area be prepared prior to the shaping treatment?

4 How can you minimise client discomfort during the eyebrow shaping treatment?

5 What after care advice should you give to a client following an eyebrow shaping treatment?

6 What hygiene and safety precautions should be followed when performing an eyebrow shape?

7 Name four contra indications that would prevent a permanent tinting treatment from being carried out.

8 If a model complains of irritation during an eyelash tinting treatment, what action would you take?

9 For how long would you allow the tint to process when treating a model with (a) blond hair? and (b) red hair?

10 When should eyelash perming not be recommended?

chapter 7

Make-up basics

This chapter will explain the make-up techniques for the application of the various types of make-up available. It will cover individual aspects of the face, looks for eyes, eyebrows, lips, cheeks, etc., which will be referred to when compiling total looks later in this chapter and subsequent chapters. This is probably the most important chapter in the book. Learning basic application techniques thoroughly in the early days of your training will set you up for a great career.

Learning objectives

In this chapter you will learn about:

- **the sequence for applying make-up**
- **make-up application techniques:**
  - **foundations and concealers**
  - **powders**
  - **eye shadows and creams**
  - **eyeliners and eyebrow products**
  - **lip colours and gloss**
  - **highlighters and shaders**
  - **blushers and bronzers**
- **application and completed looks for age ranges post 16, post 35 and post 55**
- **make-up for people wearing spectacles**
- **make-up for redheads**
- **a special occasion – an Asian wedding**

THE SEQUENCE OF APPLYING MAKE-UP

There are no hard and fast rules for applying make-up in any set order, there are many different sequences, all of which work well. What is important is to remember the final look you are aiming for, and to apply the make-up in a logical order, one that fits the look.

One example of a sequence for applying make-up might be as follows:

- cleanse, tone and moisturise – using products suitable for your model's skin
- foundation
- concealer
- eyebrows
- eyes
- lips
- powder
- powder blusher and highlighting
- contouring – shading

Another sequence might be:

- cleanse, tone and moisturise – using products suitable for your model's skin
- neutralisers and concealers
- foundation
- powder
- highlighting and shading
- eyes and eyebrows
- lips

There really is no right or wrong way – a good clean, finished look is your aim. There is also no rule to say that foundation has to go on first, or that it has to go on at all! For example, if you had selected to do a smoky eye look, would you really want to spend ages getting the foundation just right, only to leave specks of eye colour on the cheek area? You can hold a tissue under the eye to catch falling eye shadow, and you can also apply extra powder under the eye area, to be brushed off later, taking with it any unwanted dark specks. However, it is much easier to prepare the eye areas first (see later) and concentrate on getting the eyes perfect, regardless of getting any product over the cheeks. Once the eyes are perfect, you can wipe off any excess over the cheeks, and then apply foundation. You end up with a really clean look. There is nothing worse than fantastic eyes spoiled by grey cheeks where excess eye shadow has fallen.

MAKE-UP APPLICATION TECHNIQUES FOR FOUNDATION

The many different types of foundations available are explained in Chapter 4. Applying foundation is the most important step in any make-up, as it evens out the skin tones and can hide imperfections. Foundation should match the natural skin tone exactly. Only a well-applied foundation, to the whole face, including cheeks, eyelids and lips, will give you a good base upon which to begin adding further colour. Never rush the application of foundation, as no matter how perfect you make-up the eyes or lips, or how good your highlighting and contouring is, it will all be spoiled if the foundation is the wrong colour or poorly applied.

This chapter will concentrate on the basic application of foundation for general day and evening wear, for beauty and editorial work. In the level three theatrical make-up in Chapter 11, you will apply foundation from one to three times darker than natural base skin colour, which allows for the fading of colour under strong lighting. You will also learn how to apply very light foundations, even white, to complement character make-ups.

You will need a good selection of foundations in your kit box. The minimum is six basic colours ranging from very light to very dark, from which you will be able to mix any colour you need. However, three foundations for light skins in light, medium and dark shades and three foundations for dark skins, in light, medium and dark shades, would give you an ideal range of foundations. Choose products that also provide protection against the sun's UV rays. Oil-free foundation is good for oily skins, whilst moisturising foundations are better for drier and normal skins.

There are foundation ranges specifically made for dark skins. The main difference is that these foundations contain no titanium dioxide which has a tendency to leave a grey look on dark skins.

Foundation sponges

Wedge-shaped sponges are excellent for applying foundation. Immerse them in cold water first and squeeze out most of the water before using them, or the sponge will not flow over the face, and it will hold too much product, resulting in wastage. Start at the forehead and work quickly down the face, always working downward and outward, and over the eyes and lips, because they also need foundation. Alternatively you could use specially formulated eye and lip primers as foundation on these areas (see Chapter 4).

Foundation brushes

Make-up applicator brushes (see Chapter 4) are large flat brushes ideally suited for applying liquid foundation and cream blushers. They are used in a similar manner to the wedge shaped sponges, starting at the forehead and working down and out over the face. Take care that the edges around the jaw line are blended well. If you have chosen the right colour you should see no hard lines.

Applying foundation with either a foundation brush or wedge-shaped sponges

1 Cleanse, tone and moisturise using appropriate products to suit your model's skin.
2 Observe the model's face colour and compare it to the colour of her arms and torso. Your aim is that the face and neck should look as if they are part of the same person! Some models use a fake tan on their bodies but not on their face or vice versa – ideally the face and the body should be the same colour.

> **TIP**
>
> If you apply a foundation coloured concealer first, there is every chance you will wipe it off with the sponge when applying the base foundation, and therefore it makes sense to apply it *after* the foundation, which can also conceal – so less concealer is needed. Neutralisers on the other hand – the lilac, green and peach colours used for neutralising blues, reds and yellows must be applied *under* the base foundation.

> **HEALTH AND SAFETY**
>
> Good habits start early – always mix foundations on a palette – not on the back of your hand.

3 Choose the right colour for your model, either by choosing a single colour, or by mixing different colours together on a palette. Test on the side of the face/jaw line. With practice you will be able to do this quite quickly, as you learn to observe skin colours and get to know the colours in your make-up kit. Once you have the right colour, use either a sponge or a brush and start to apply the product from the top, working downwards and outwards – try to work quite quickly. Some water-based products dry quickly and can leave streak marks.

4 If you are not using a specific primer for the eyes and lips, then take the foundation right over these areas.

5 Take care to avoid the eyebrows and sides of the face where fine hair may be growing. You should use a cosmetic bud to blend foundation into these areas.

MAKE-UP APPLICATION TECHNIQUES FOR CONCEALER

HEALTH AND SAFETY

Lipstick concealers – never apply these directly from the original container. Take a little product with a spatula and place it on a palette, then, using a lip brush, apply directly to the skin.

A concealer's job is to conceal blemishes – so do not get confused with concealers and colour correctors, which even out the skin's undertones. If your product is white, pink, greasy, dry, chalky, too pale or too dark, it may emphasise the very flaws you are trying to hide. The concealer colour should be a similar colour to the foundation. You can mix a little concealer, which has a heavier consistency than foundation, with the foundation you used to make the colour a better match and easier and lighter to apply. Using an appropriately sized brush, cover the blemish with concealer (not colour corrector), blending out towards the edges. Concealer can be applied before or after foundation. Applying the concealer *before* the foundation, you can see every blemish which is advantageous, but when you apply foundation after the concealer it may disturb the concealing product. By concealing *after* foundation, the foundation may have done enough to conceal the majority of the blemishes so less concealer will be needed. You can concentrate on the small imperfections the foundation did not cover. There is no right or wrong way; the most important aspect is that the colours of the concealer and foundation match.

Powder

Professional make-up artists usually use a loose translucent powder, which will not change the colour of the foundation you have carefully chosen or specially mixed. Apply using a large powder brush. Put a little product into the lid of the powder container and take it from there, avoiding taking too much product on the brush. Tap off any excess powder and brush lightly over the face, starting at the top and working in a downwards and outwards motion. You may decide to use a coloured powder – a face bronzer for example. Remember that the face should be the same colour as the body.

MAKE-UP APPLICATION TECHNIQUES FOR EYEBROWS

Eyebrows are often overlooked, but as the eyebrows frame the face, they should be defined for a completed make-up look. Instructions for how to re-shape eyebrows can be found in Chapter 6. However, you can also enhance the eyebrow using make-up.

Take care when drawing in brows with a pencil as this can make them look hard or even 'cartoonish'. Eye shadow or an eyebrow shadow in a tone that matches your hair colour is the most natural way to fill in and enhance eyebrows.

What shade should you use?

Many students, when they first start out, will simply choose 'brown' for eyebrow enhancing for everybody! However, whilst brown may indeed suit many people, the colour to choose depends to a large extent upon hair colour.

Hair colour	Brow colour
Pale blond	Light ash blond
Medium to dark blond	Ash blond to sable
Light to medium brown	Sable to mahogany
Medium to dark brown	Mahogany to reddish brown
Black	Mahogany to smoke (never charcoal or black)
Light red	Taupe or camel
Medium red	Taupe or camel
Dark red	Reddish brown
Slate	Mahogany or dark grey
Light grey	Slate or grey
White	Grey or taupe

Darkening the eyebrows

The eyebrows may have a good shape but just be too fair. Check the guidelines in Chapter 6 to ascertain where the brows should start and finish. Marking with a white eye pencil will help you. Choose an eyebrow powder or eyebrow pencil to complement the hair colour – see above. If you are unsure, you can choose a lighter colour first – it is easier to add product and make the eyebrows darker than to remove product to make them lighter – and eyebrows take colour very well.

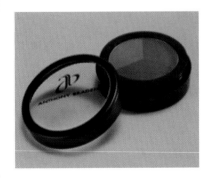

A trio of eyebrow colours – Anthony Braden Cosmetics

Using brush and powder

Brush the eyebrows into shape using a brow brush. Work upwards and outwards to give the brow more definition and help to open up the whole eye area. Using a small pointed brush or firm flat and angled brush, take a small amount of powder, lightly tap off the excess, and, starting from the inside, brush onto the hairs in the direction of hair growth with a feathering action. Work over the natural shape of the brow, darkening as you go, and accentuating the arch by brushing some colour along the upper edge of the brow.

Using an eye shadow or a brow powder gives the brows a softer, more natural look than using pencils.

Using an eyebrow pencil

Choose a colour that is not too dark – your aim is to enhance, unless you want to make the eyebrows the focal point of a particular look – a Groucho Marx for example! Starting from the inside, draw small angled lines over the natural brow, just enough to emphasise the brow.

Fill in sparse eyebrows

Using the same technique as above, choose a colour similar to the eyebrow's natural colour and, using a small pointed brush or firm angled brush, or a pencil, fill in the gaps.

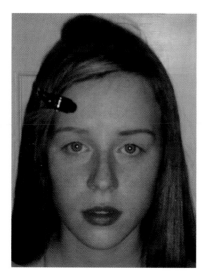

Defining the eyebrows – before (left) and after (right)

Create eyebrows

You may need to create eyebrows if:

- you have blanked them out with wax (Chapter 11) in order to create a particular look
- your model has no eyebrows due to illness
- your model has no eyebrows due to over tweezing throughout the years

A consultation with the model is needed to ascertain the size and shape of brows she requires. Having decided on the size and shape to suit the model, and using the guidelines described in Chapter 6, mark where the brows will begin and end, using a white pencil. You may use an eyebrow stencil if this will help you to get both eyebrows exactly the same. Showing your model the different style of stencils helps her with the choice of shapes available. If you have no stencils, then draw a shape for her. Much will depend on the model's features – her face shape, the width of her eyes, etc. An eyebrow pencil is better than powder when creating eyebrows. Choose a light colour first and complete the shape on the model. When you and the model are satisfied that the size and shapes are correct, you can darken with eyebrow make-up to match her hair colour and complexion and the overall look you are trying to achieve.

Re-creating eyebrows

Eyebrows are rarely identical, but for photographic work they need to be as similar as possible. To re-create uneven brows, it is often easier to make a small change to each brow than drastic changes to one.

If a model were to have one curved brow and one brow with a high arch, you could draw in a small arch on the curved brow, and reduce the arch on the arched brow, possibly by blanking out with foundation.

TIP ✔

Eyebrows fade as you get older. The solution is not to darken them too much. The older the model, the lighter your touch needs to be when applying eyebrow products. Don't forget to check the end result in daylight to make sure you have a natural, finished look

STUDENT ACTIVITY

7.1 Re-creating eyebrows – become aware of people's eyebrows. Look at the eyebrows of friends, family and colleagues (both male and female). If any of them have irregular eyebrows, ask if you can practice re-creating them. Take before and after photographs at each attempt, to record your progress.

MAKE-UP APPLICATION TECHNIQUES FOR EYE SHADOWS AND CREAMS

Natural eye make-up

There are many ways to apply eye make-up for day and evening wear – natural, light and pearly, dark and dramatic, matt or iridescent – the choices are endless. Here we look at some basic looks for eyes using powder shadows.

The rule regarding eye shadow is that when you look at a made-up face, you should see the *eyes* and not the eye shadow! The general rule is that light shades bring out eyes, darker shades give them dimension. If a model has small eyes, you may want to stay with lighter shades. If your client has large or protruding eyes, use darker shades.

Before starting any eye make-up using powder eye shadows, the eye lid area must be prepared. This can either be achieved by applying the foundation colour over the eye lids and then applying powder to set. Alternatively you can use an eye primer. An eye primer is a specially formulated product that helps retain the colour of eye shadow and therefore keeps the eye make-up on longer. It is a two-in-one product in that it covers like a foundation but dries as if it were powdered.

If using cream eye shadows, the preparation of the eyelid is different. With a powder eye shadow, you apply a foundation colour and lightly dust with a powder before adding the coloured shadow. When using a cream, you use a primer, or apply to unpowdered foundation. A light dusting of translucent powder may be applied after the cream shadow, to set.

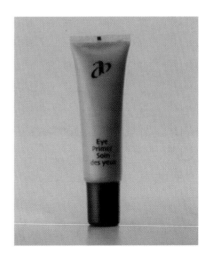

Eye primer by Anthony Braden Cosmetics

A two-tone simple day make-up

This is a fast and easy way to use two colours of eye shadow for everyday use.

1 Having prepared the eye area, start by choosing two colours – one medium and one light. Apply the light colour over the whole lid. This could be a beige colour.

2 Taking the darker colour, which could be a medium brown, green or grey, apply to the lower lid only.

3 Blend the two colours together with a blending brush so no hard lines are showing.

4 Apply a little of the medium colour under the lashes if desired. How far you go under the lashes towards the inner edge would depend upon the size and shape of the eye. Get right under the lashes, leaving no white areas of skin uncovered between the lashes and the eye colour.

5 Complete with brown mascara.

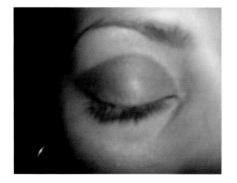

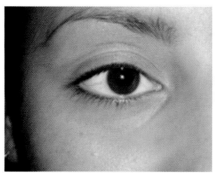

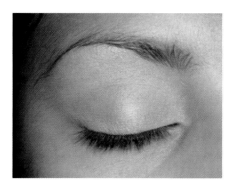

Two tone day make-up – before

Stage 1 – preparation of area – concealer under eye, primer over eyelid

Stage 2 – apply light colour to whole area

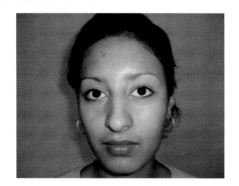

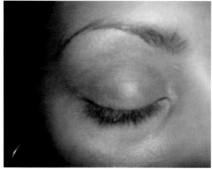

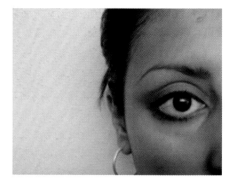

Stage 3 – apply second colour to lower lid

Stage 4 – blend the two colours together

Stage 5 – two tone day make-up – final look

TIP	
By darkening the make-up you will make it more distinctive and will turn a day look into an evening look.	

The triangle

1 Having prepared the eye area, start by choosing two colours – one medium and one dark, and apply the medium colour over the whole lid.

2 Ask the model to close her eyes. Draw in a triangle shape with the dark colour. First, find the socket line by using gentle pressure with an eye shadow brush, above the lid. The socket line provides one edge of the triangle, the eyelashes provide the second. The third should be no further across the eye than one third.

3 Once the shape has been defined, fill in with the dark colour.

4 Blend to take away the hard third edge, but retain an obvious triangle shape.

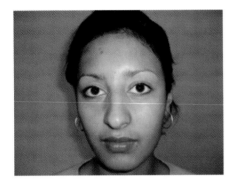 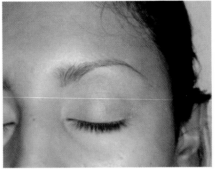 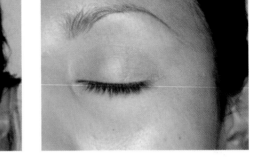

Triangle look – before

Stages 1 and 2 – apply medium colour to whole lid. Draw in triangle shape using dark colour

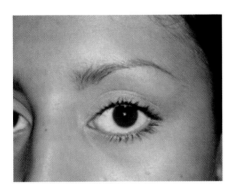

Stage 3 – completed triangle look using Black by Design Make-up

TIP	✔
To ensure eyes are the same, it is recommended to work on both eyes at once – Stage 1 on both eyes, followed by Stage 2 on both eyes, etc.	

Socket lines

1 Having prepared the eye area, choose three colours to suit the model – one medium/natural shade, one dark shade and one light shade to highlight. Apply the natural shade over the entire eye area. Choose a colour that will show up for the socket area.

2 Using a small brush, find the socket line with the eyes open. The model should then close her eye to enable you to draw in a line of dark colour. Blend well. Iridescent colours work well with this look. Do not make the line too close to the inner edge and don't work too far up or too far down.

3 Apply highlighter to under the brow area.

4 Use shadow to draw in eyeliner, if necessary, using a small brush. Using a shadow instead of a pencil will stay on longer.

5 Complete the look by using black mascara.

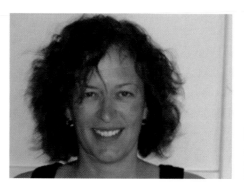

Socket line look before

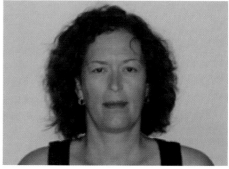

Stage 1 – prepare eyes, conceal under eye area and apply natural shade over whole eye

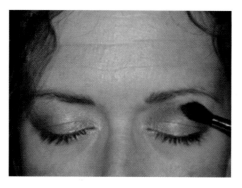

Stage 2 – define socket line with dark colour, and blend well

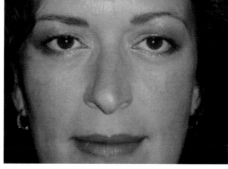

Stages 3, 4 and 5 – final look well blended using three colours

TIP	

No-one to practise on? No excuse! You can practise any of the eye looks on yourself. Only with continued practice will you become fully competent.

Cat eye

As you can see from the illustrations, this is a very dramatic look, which drags the eyes upward like a cat. It is often used in fashion shows – on the catwalk obviously!

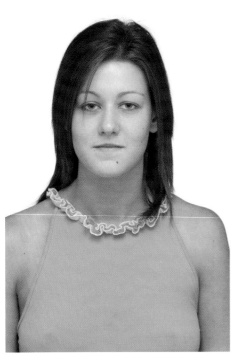

Cat eyes – before

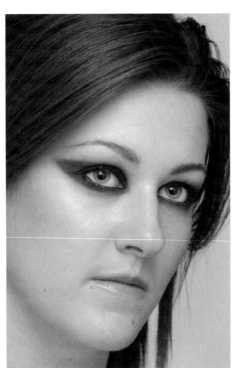

Cat eyes – after

Long eye

This method of eye make-up is used on eyes that are close together, and the illusion of them being further apart is desired.

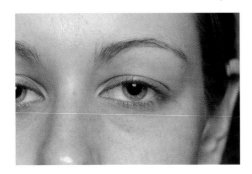

Long eye – before

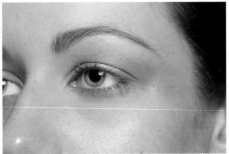

Long eye – after

Smoky eye

The smoky eye is very popular at present and suits most eyes. Browns and black/charcoal are popular colours for this look, but experiment with other colours too.

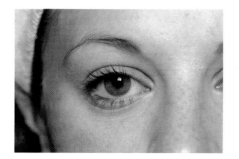

Smoky eye – before

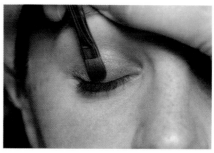

Stage 1 – apply colour to eyelid

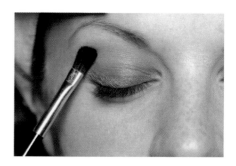

Stage 2 – blend to just above the socket line

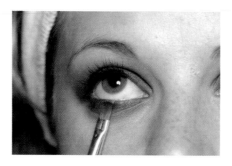

Stage 3 – take colour under lower lashes blending well

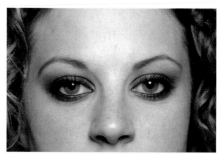

Final look – perfectly blended smoky eye look

Contemporary editorial look

This look derives from the smoky eye, but has been made more dramatic with the application of eyeliner and cloggy mascara.

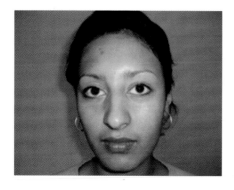

Contemporary editorial look – before

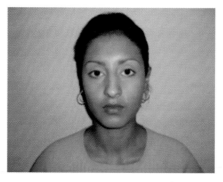

Stage 1 – apply concealer under eye area and prepare eye area using foundation and powder or eye primer

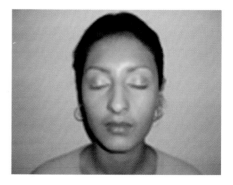

Stage 2 – apply colour over eyelid area

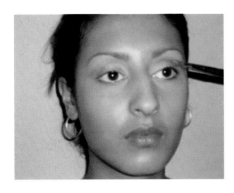

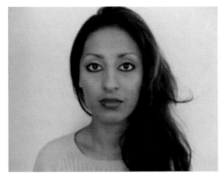

Stage 3 – colour can be applied with eyes open to just above socket line to get a perfect, even finish to both eyes

Stage 4 – blend well, apply eyeliner and mascara. Contemporary editorial look – final

These are six classic eye make-ups; two-tone, triangle, socket lines, cats eye, long eye and smoky eye, but the possibilities are endless. Once you have mastered the above techniques, experiment and create your own designs.

Softeners using strong colours

The emphasis of this Asian wedding eye make-up is on colour and shape. Three distinct colours have been used – two strong colours and a highlighter, with eyeliner and mascara added for definition. The end result is a beautiful make-up using strong colour but creating a soft bridal look.

STUDENT ACTIVITY

7.2   Use your colours! Do not practise just your favourite looks with browns and neutral colours. Practise with every colour in your make-up kit, every look, over and over again.

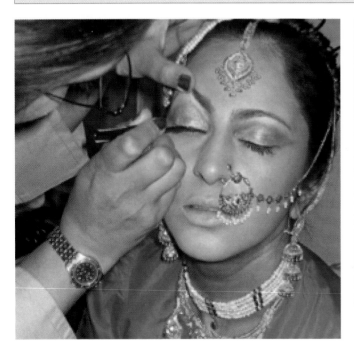

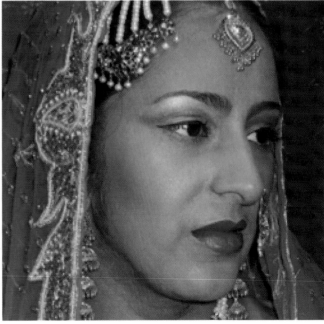

Asian bride applying eyeliner

Asian bride eye make-up – final

MAKE-UP APPLICATION TECHNIQUES FOR LIP COLOURS

Lip liners, colours and gloss

Lip liners are used:

- to define lips
- to avoid the lipstick seeping out onto the skin – known as 'bleeding'
- to assist lip colour to last longer.

The trend at the time of writing this book, for general make-up use, is not to use lip liner, or to use a lip liner in the same colour as the main lip colour. An obvious line between your lip liner and lip colour is not only dated, it can be unflattering. If you choose to use a lip liner, for the most natural look, pick a liner that is the same shade or *one* shade darker than your natural lip colour. Traditionally, lip liners have always been applied first. This is still usually the case, but there is nothing stopping you from applying lip liner *after* applying your colour.

If the model has even lips, always follow the natural lip line when using lip liner pencils. You may then want to use a lip brush to soften and blend the liner, on the inside edge. If you have small lips, don't try to create the illusion of bigger ones by drawing outside your lip line; the best way to enhance them is with a medium tone lipstick or a creamy gloss.

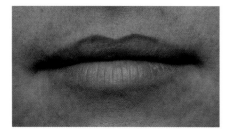
Stage 1 – Cupid's bow top

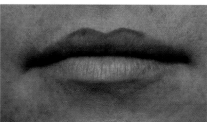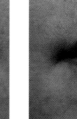
Stage 2 – Cupid's bow bottom

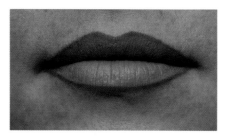
Stage 3 – outline complete

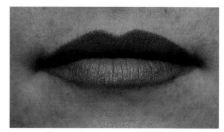
Filled in with light colour – wrong

Filled in with same colour – right

Always use a lip brush to apply the main lip colour. For a selection of lip colours see Chapter 8. This section also shows you how the lip 'colours' look in black and white photographs, where the 'colour' used is not as important as the 'shade'.

Lip gloss is used to give shine to lips and is applied in the same way as lip colour, with a brush. If no lip gloss is available, use a little Vaseline for the same effect.

MAKE-UP ARTIST PROFILE: JUDIE BECQUE

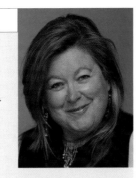

How and when did you start in the business?

In 2001 my daughter went to Disneyland to dance and there was no one to do the make-up. I just got involved and loved it.

Was there a turning point in your career?

Yes, when people started trusting my judgement and I was allowed to design my own looks.

What do you consider to be important qualities for a make-up artist?

Look and listen to what people want. Always help your model to feel relaxed and enjoy the experience.

What is your most memorable/exciting/best paid job?

When I first did a job for a very famous group of hairdressers and they said 'We trust you. Do what you want! Oh and don't forget Sky TV will be filming you!'

Have you had any disasters?

Not disasters as such, just not putting foundation on the eyes and then expecting the bright yellow I was using to show up – it didn't.

What advice would you give to young people entering the industry?

Always listen, you might think you know everything – you don't. I still learn from every job I do.

In your experience, would you advise those training to become make-up artists to specialise in one area only, or to gain experience, through Continued Professional Development courses (CPD) in many different areas of make-up?

I would do a general course in hair and make-up, then I personally found I enjoyed one particular area, so I went and found another course that specialised in that area and now I thoroughly enjoy every job I get.

MAKE-UP APPLICATION TECHNIQUES FOR HIGHLIGHTERS AND SHADERS

Where to highlight and where to contour depends on face shape, size and colouring. As a general rule, highlighters enhance features, shading detracts from features.

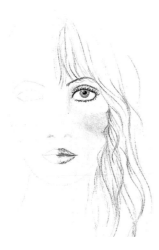

Oval face with highlighter to enhance features

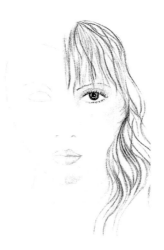

Heart face with shading, lessening the width at the top of the head.

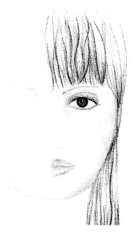

Round face using highlighter and shading colours to 'lengthen' appearance of face

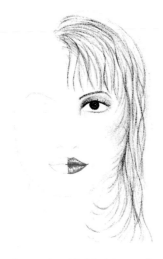

Square face using highlighter and shading colours to soften features

STUDENT ACTIVITY

7.3   Draw an oblong face and a triangular face shape in the same format as the basic five face shapes.

An oblong face would need shading under the jawline and on forehead to 'shorten' features, whereas a triangular face would need shading to temples to lessen width and to soften features.

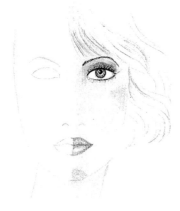

Long – shading needed to top and bottom and sides to achieve a more oval look.

BLUSHERS AND BRONZERS

Make-up fashions change and in Chapter 8 you will learn that, throughout the eras, women have desired to change their natural skin colour. At present it is fashionable to have a 'sun kissed' look, without damaging the skin from UV rays. Therefore, blushers and bronzers come in a huge range and can be applied virtually anywhere over the face and body. But be careful to match all exposed skin. A 'tanned' face with white décolletage will look unsightly. When applying powdered blushers and bronzers, use the largest brush in your kit. Cream products can be applied using sponges. Always tap off excess product before applying to the skin.

APPLICATION AND COMPLETED LOOKS FOR AGE RANGES POST 16, POST 35 AND POST 55

Age range: post 16

The teenage years is the time to start looking after your skin. Sunscreen is probably the best investment anyone can make at this time. Clients in this age group will need a good cleanser, eye cream, a tinted moisturiser and a concealer, and the minimum of make-up during the day. However, now is the time when clients want to follow trends and experiment. The illustrations here show a contemporary evening look with the emphasis on the eye make-up, and a look called Fresh and Freckles, which, although it looks like a totally unmade-up face, is in fact a full make-up including the freckles!

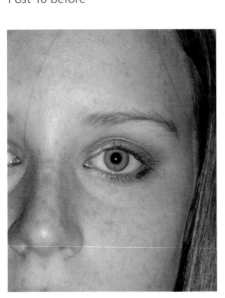

Post 16 before

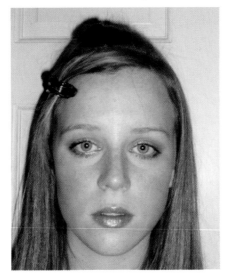

Stage 1 – light foundation and concealer enhance the eyebrows

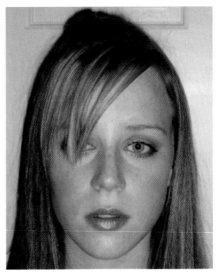

Stage 2 – apply predominant eye colour

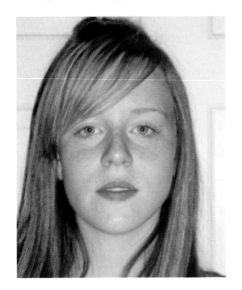

Stage 3 – add further colours to eye make-up

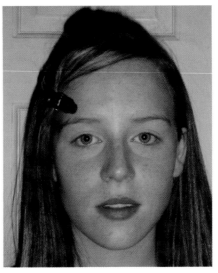

Stage 4 – apply eyeliner, mascara and lip gloss

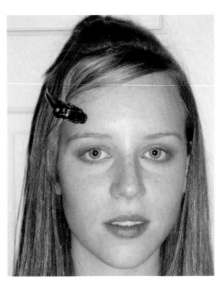

Post 16 final look

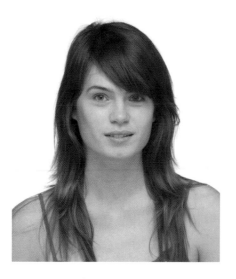

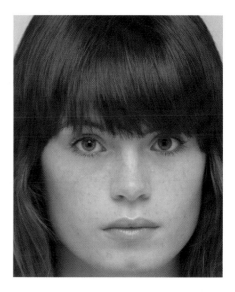

Post 16 – before – Fresh and freckles

Post 16 – after – Fresh and freckles

TIP	
To make freckles – take a well sharpened brown eyebrow pencil and gently flick freckles onto appropriate areas of the face. For fashion make-up it is imperative that these look 'natural'.	

Age range: post 35

The area around the eyes will start getting noticeably drier and lined among this age group, so care must be taken when applying concealers, as they tend to sit in these lines. Apply all make-up carefully, choosing products that will protect and nourish the skin. Women of this age range have had time to experiment, and make mistakes, and should therefore by now be confident with their make-up, knowing well what suits them.

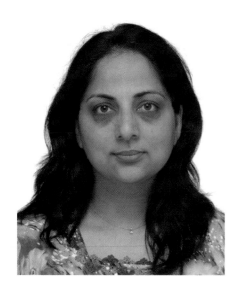

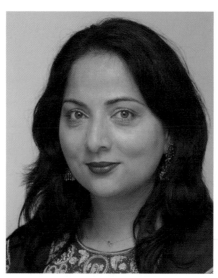

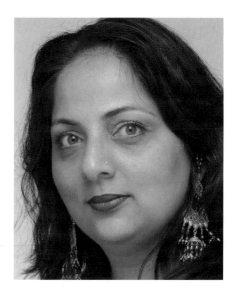

Asian lady post 35 – before

Asian lady post 35 – example 1

Asian lady post 35 – example 2

Age range: post 55

Among clients in this age group, loss of eyebrow colour will be evident and therefore shaping and defining the brows is essential as part of their daily make-up routine. Preparation of the skin is of particular importance for this age range. Many companies have light moisturisers with 'lifting' capabilities for application under foundation. These moisturisers gently lighten the skin, making the foundation easier to apply and greatly enhances the make-up. A touch of blusher will give the face a lift, and lining the lips is recommended as 'bleeding' often occurs with this age range. Attention to detail is important as is an appreciation of the model's overall look.

TIP
A good phrase to remember for this age group is 'less is more'. The heavier you make the make-up, the older the client will look, so be sparing in all applications.

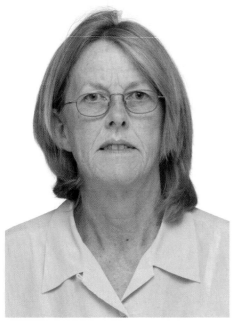

Post 55 lady before

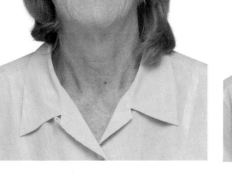

Post 55 lady after

Make-up for people who wear spectacles

The appearance of the eyes alters depending upon the function of the model's lenses. If a model is short sighted, the lenses will make the eye appear smaller, therefore select brighter, lighter colours. If the model is long sighted, the lenses will magnify her eyes, so make-up should be more subtle. Avoid frosted colours and lash building mascaras.

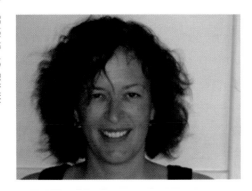

Spectacles before

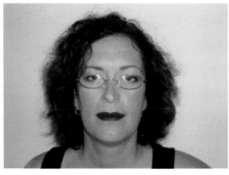

Gold frames – a less dramatic eye to enhance more gentle frame – emphasis on the lips

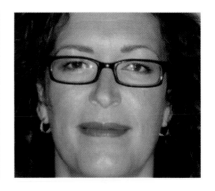

Dark frames – good use of eyeliner and mascara – enabling you to still see the eyes. A balanced make-up

Make-up for red heads

With a sensational hair colour, natural or otherwise, redheads can look striking with dramatic make-up or beautifully natural with subtle make-up. The photos illustrate how a beautiful natural make-up is applied to a red head.

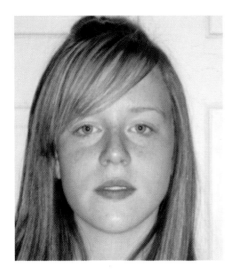

Before picture for redhead

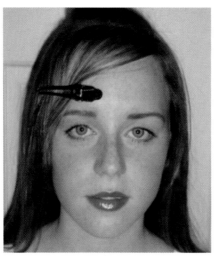

Apply light tinted foundation, medium colour on eyes with brown eye liner, mascara and lip gloss. Don't forget to enhance eyebrows.

SPECIAL OCCASION – AN ASIAN WEDDING

Asian weddings are a joy to behold when it comes to make-up and colour. Traditional colours are reds and gold, with perfect foundation, unlike a British wedding where minimalist natural make-up is traditional. Refer to Chapter 14 for a more in-depth look at the traditions of face and body decoration.

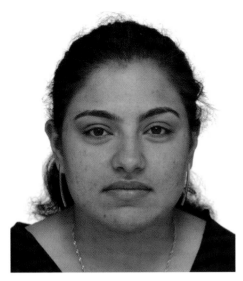

Asian bride before

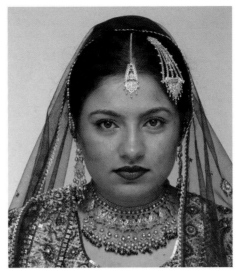

Asian bride after

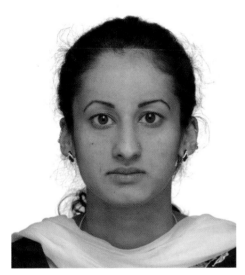

Asian bridesmaid before

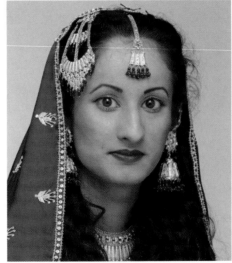

Asian bridesmaid after

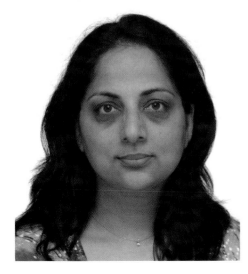

Wedding guest before

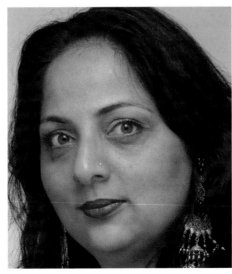

Wedding guest after

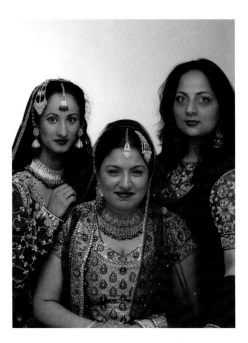

Group photo

Assessment of knowledge and understanding

Knowledge review

1 Give an example of a sequence for applying make-up.

2 Give one instance when foundation should be applied after eye shadow.

3 What product could be used as an alternative to foundation around the eye or lip area?

4 What size brush should be used for applying bronzer?

5 When might you need to create eyebrows?

6 Which shape of eyes would most benefit from the 'long eye' look?

7 Why are lip liners used?

8 What is the best way to create the illusion of bigger lips?

9 What are the alternatives to lip gloss, if there is none available?

10 How will eyes appear on a person wearing lenses for long sightedness?

chapter 8

Fashion and photographic make-up

Fashion make-up artists need to be constantly up to date with all the latest colours, products and looks, and their work must be of the highest standard, as the majority of it will be photographed for prestigious magazines and events. Fashion work includes editorial and advertising, fashion shows, music videos and catalogue photography. Your work may therefore appear on the front cover of *Glamour*, *Vogue* or *Harpers & Queen*, on the latest pop video, or seen by millions in London, Milan, Paris or New York at their prestigious fashion weeks, where the make-up is almost as important as the clothes! Although not as prestigious as fashion or editorial work, working for catalogue companies can be very well paid. Each style of work comes with its own technical differences, which will be covered in this chapter. Read Chapter 15, 'Career options', for more information on working in this area.

Learning objectives

In this chapter you will learn about:

- **photographic make-up**

- **make-up through the centuries**

- **basic make-up for a man**

- **fashion looks**
  - **editorial**
  - **catwalks, fashion shows and pop videos**
  - **catalogues**

PHOTOGRAPHIC MAKE-UP

Choosing the right colours to suit the occasion and the make-up will come with practice. If you are applying make-up for a black and white photograph, you need to look beyond the *colours* you are applying to the

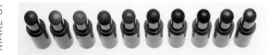

Assorted lip colours by Anthony Braden Cosmetics

model, and think about the shades. Practice *seeing* the final black and white image you are trying to create in your mind. The following conversion table for lip colour will help you – notice how the *colour* becomes irrelevant, but the *shade* is apparent. Notice too the perfect application of the product which is needed for photographic work because the camera picks up every detail. The lip colour is applied to the very edges of the natural lip line with no edges left uncoloured.

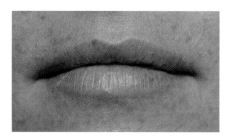

Nude lips

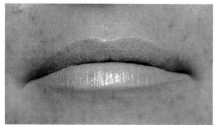

Solar Flare

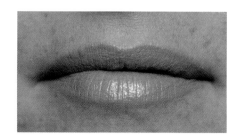

Soul

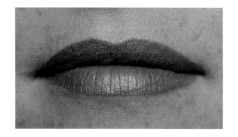

Calliope

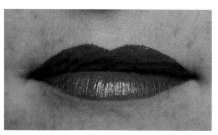

Sea Crush

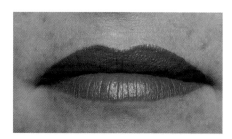

Rose

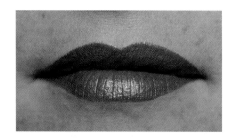

Oxygen

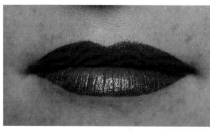

Calgary Flame

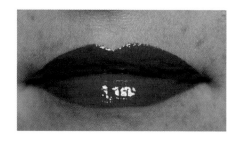

Lounge

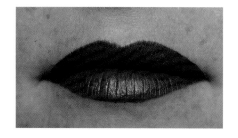

18K Gold

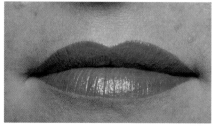

Wine

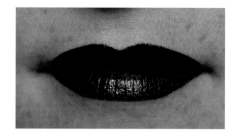

Black

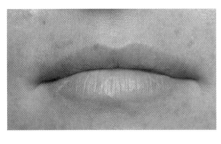

Nude lips

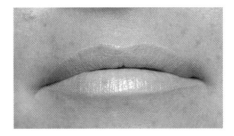

Solar flare

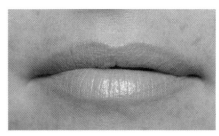

Soul

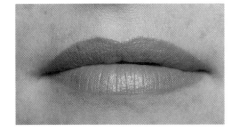

Calliope

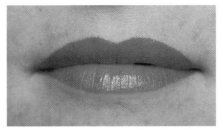

Sea Crush

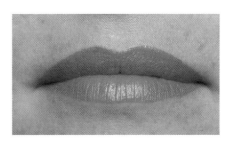

Rose

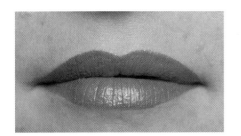

Oxygen

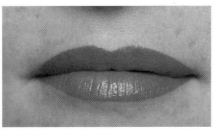

Calgary Flame

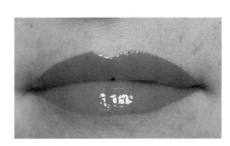

Lounge

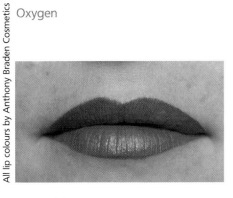

18K Gold

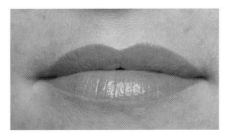

Wine

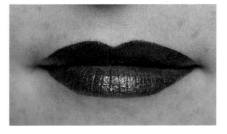

Black

All lip colours by Anthony Braden Cosmetics

Even when you are applying make-up for colour photography, which will probably be most of the time, always keep in mind what the make-up will look like as a black and white print. When doing test shoots, ask the photographer for black and white prints as well as colour prints for your portfolio. Should you subsequently be asked to apply make-up for a black and white print, you will have a much better idea of what your colours/shades will look like.

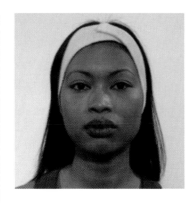

Before make-up

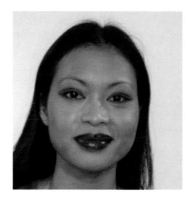

Popular smoky eye make-up
with Anthony Braden 'Lounge'
lipstick

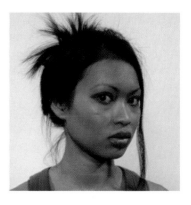

Lip shade changed to Anthony
Braden 'Wine'

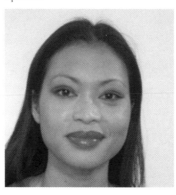

The 'Lounge' lipstick shade was
chosen purposely to create this
shade in a black and white
photo

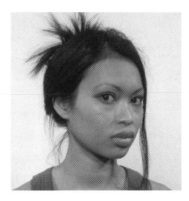

The 'wine' lipstick shade was
chosen purposely to create this
shade in a black and white
photo

TIP

Although taking your own photographs is not as professional as having them done by a
professional photographer, it is a good idea to invest in either a digital or a Polaroid camera.
You can then take photographs of all your work for your college portfolio. With cameras
nowadays, you can choose whether to have prints produced in colour or in black and white,
and it is a real learning experience to see your work in both.

MAKE-UP THROUGH THE CENTURIES

Students often ask why learning basic make-up application is not sufficient
training and they cannot understand the need to learn about the make-up
of past eras. Be assured that all modern make-up has its roots in the past.
At the time of writing this text, a strong 1950s influence was returning in
fashion and make-up practices. Fashion shows, pop videos and catwalk work
often have a theme – this could be absolutely anything from designing an
eighteenth-century punk make-up to being required to make-up someone
with 1950s eyes (taking the eyeliner into a flick) with 1920s lips (cupid's
bow), or could have a more modern 1960s influence. You need to be aware

of the main features of each look. You may be asked to re-create a look on the day you turn up for a shoot with no time to research it. In fact, some full-time theatrical and media make-up courses require a qualification in history and art as an entry requirement.

Seventeenth-century make-up looks

'Foundations' were being used as early, if not earlier, than the seventeenth century. Although during this century fashions altered, we traditionally remember seventeenth-century make-up as a white powdered base. To contrast with the white foundation (to make it look whiter) and due to some unsightly skin disorders of the day, it became fashionable to disguise imperfections with black taffeta or leather patches shaped as stars, half-moons and circles.

Eighteenth-century make-up looks

The white powdered and black patched 'look' continued into the eighteenth century. To ladies of fashion, make-up was essential, and as the century progressed they used more and more of it. Women tended to pencil their eyebrows high and thin, touch up their veins with blue (to give the illusion of being 'blue blooded' aristocrats) and they applied abundant amounts of rouge. The lips were small and rosebud shaped and painted red. The overall look appeared almost theatrical, especially from our modern viewpoint.

Nineteenth-century make-up looks

During this century only stage actors and courtesans openly applied make-up and ordinary women wore cosmetics very discreetly. When Queen Victoria (1837–1901) came to the British throne there was a complete reaction against the use of any paint on the face. Women continued to use cosmetics but, since this was now considered vulgar, they had to use even more discretion. Many cosmetics were home made. Officially, powder, creams, and lotions were all that were used.

Twentieth-century make-up history and looks

Unlike the previous two centuries, when the trend was to over paint the face, in the twentieth century women started to use cosmetics and make-up to enhance particular features. The century started with Queen Victoria still on the throne of England and women doing little to adorn themselves. During the early years of the twentieth century, rouge was the main item of make-up, but gradually other new revolutionary items appeared. Nail polishes came on the market in 1907 and new powders and foundations were being formulated with a choice of colours. The beauty secrets of the day involved a clean skin, plenty of rest, an 'eye-cup' (for salt water eye baths), a pair of tweezers, an eyelash ointment and cold cream.

The 1920s

The women of the 1920s wanted their lives to be different after the strict morals of the Victorian era, so they drank alcohol, smoked cigarettes and started to wear make-up abundantly – something only previously done by 'loose women'! Rouge, powder, eyeliner and lipstick became extremely popular. Make-up can change quite a lot within the ten years of each decade. Fashions in clothes and make-up tend to change annually – although there are strong main features that do last for much longer. Foundation colours, for example, changed several times during the 1920s. In the early years of this decade, cream and ivory shades were popular, followed closely by peachy shades. The middle years tended to see more natural shades. By the end of the decade, foundation colours tended to be one shade lighter than the natural skin tone, and that is the way we usually recreate a 1920s make-up today. The other main feature was the small, perfectly shaped lips, known as the cupid's bow. You may need to block out natural lips at the outer corners to make the lips appear smaller. Hair fashions also underwent dramatic changes during the 1920s. Young women cut their previously long hair into a style called the 'Bob', because it looked masculine. This was eventually replaced by an even shorter hair cut called the 'Shingle' or 'Eaton cut'. The Shingle cut was slicked down and had a curl on each side of the face that covered the woman's ears. Women often completed the look with a felt, bell shaped hat called a Cloche. At the end of the 1920s, the stock market crashed and the world was plunged into what is known as the Great Depression. Frivolity and recklessness were forced to come to an end – however, the new 'free woman' remained.

Main features of 1920s make-up

- Foundation   pale and powdered
- Eyebrows   long and thin (you may need to block out originals first, see Chapter 11)
- Eyes   smoky, black, soft and smudgy
- Lips   cupid's bow – true red
- Cheeks   gentle pink blusher applied to the apple of the cheek
- Overall look sad wistful expression

Re-creating a 1920s look

Look carefully at the face you are going to make-up. Do the eyebrows need shaping, changing or blocking out? You may decide you want to do this preparation work before applying foundation to avoid spoiling the foundation later.

1 Have everything ready.

2 Cleanse, tone and moisturise the skin.

3 Apply foundation to the face, one shade paler than the natural skin tone.

4 Eyebrows – straighten/darken/shape as necessary, aiming for a thin straight line.

5 Eyes – a gentle smoky eye is needed, using 'soft' blacks or browns applied to the lid area, and under the bottom lashes to create a 'circle'.

6 Lips – choose a true red lip liner and draw the required shape. Then apply colour with a lip brush. You may need to camouflage the outer corners to get the required shape. The lip 'rouge' was applied heavily and then blotted.

7 With a pink cream blusher, apply to apple of cheeks and blend edges, to give a natural glow.

8 Using translucent powder, powder over the cheeks and nose to set the foundation (or use a powder puff if you want to be authentic).

TIP	

When creating a 1920s make-up don't get carried away with iridescent or frosted products, as they did not exist then! Historically, the cupid's bow was formed using lip rouge on the fingertip and lip liners were not used. However, to re-create a perfect cupid's bow a lip liner may be necessary.

EQUIPMENT AND PRODUCT LIST

Equipment and products for a 1920s make-up look

Equipment

Full make-up kit and brushes

Products

Pale foundation

Red lipstick

Eyebrow-shaping products

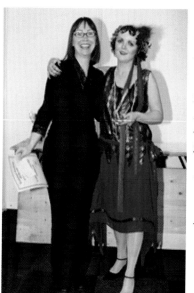

Image courtesy of Professional Beauty, Olympia 2003

1920s competition winner Olympia

The 1930s

Rouge for the cheeks and powder were the main make-up products in the early 1930s, as lipsticks and mascara went into decline after the frivolous 1920s. Many women were still highly influenced by the long deceased Queen Victoria's moral standards.

The products of the day were made by Coty, Elizabeth Arden, Maybelline, Houbigant, Revlon and of course Helena Rubinstein – all still available today, almost 80 years later. Helena Rubinstein, who started making cosmetics in Australia in 1902, in much the same way as Anita Roddick (Body Shop) did in the early 1980s, moved her business to London to expand. Her trademark was, and still is, purity of product. She considered powder to be of primary importance in any make-up and the most indispensable item on the 1930s dressing table. But it had to be extremely fine ('sifted many times through the finest silk cloth') and suited to one's type of skin. She would be aware of the fashion trends of Paris, Vienna and Rome and introduced their ideas to

English women when she thought the time was right. Whilst white, or very pale powder was still being used in England, darker powders were being used in other European cities, as it was thought this gave a healthy look and made the teeth appear whiter – much the same as we think today. It took 40 years for the healthy 'bronzed' look to come to England with the arrival of 'Charlie's Angels' in the 1970s.

Helena Rubinstein introduced compact and cream rouge, which eventually replaced the hard to apply liquid that was previously available. For evening make-up, a little rouge was also placed on the ear lobes. She found brilliant rouge acceptable with large eyes, but not with those which were 'small, soft, and serene'. Raspberry, she found, was a safe shade for everybody, although geranium was suitable for a fair skin, brunette for the olive-skinned, and crushed rose tint for the natural woman. Tangerine, she added, was still used by a few blondes and redheads, but was otherwise 'very little in favour'.

Persian eye black was applied to both the upper and lower lids with the index finger, covered with fine linen. With the optional addition of a little eyebrow pencil, the make-up was done. It was to be removed with cold cream, followed by an **astringent**.

The most significant development in make-up in the 1930s was Max Factor's Pan Cake, the first water-soluble cake foundation. The name derived from the fact that it was a cake make-up in **panchromatic** shades for film. But as it grew in popularity for street, stage and television, the range of colours expanded to meet the demand.

To a great extent Hollywood set the make-up fashions in the 1930s and appealed directly to the desire of the average woman to look like a movie star. Another development at this time was the lip brush, used by the movie stars, and whole page advertisements appeared in *Vogue* and other magazines encouraging everyone to use a sable lip brush to apply lipstick and be like a movie star! This would have been a very expensive item in the 1930s and it was not until the 1960s that make-up brushes were widely used, when Mary Quant introduced them with her make-up range.

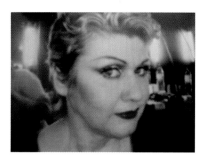

1930s look

Main features of 1930s make-up

- Foundation   porcelain base with translucent powder
- Eyebrows   concealed and re-designed in an arch shape using a pencil
- Eyes   white eye shadow over lids. Softly blended black eye shadow in socket line. Soft shadow colour may be taken underneath lower lashes (optional). Black eyeliner, dragged lengthways. Curled lashes and mascara. Add false lashes if necessary
- Lips   long full lips in a true red
- Cheeks   cream blusher blended well – colours as above
- Overall look   the sad eyed look

Recreating a 1930s look

Look carefully at the face you are going to make-up. Do the eyebrows need shaping, changing or blocking out? You may decide you want to do this preparation work before applying foundation to avoid spoiling the foundation later.

1 Have everything ready.

2 Cleanse, tone and moisturise the skin.

3 Apply foundation to the face, one shade paler than the natural skin tone and set with translucent powder.

4 Re-create the eyebrows, using a brown eyebrow pencil.

5 Apply white eye shadow to the lower lid, and black into the socket line. Apply black eyeliner and mascara.

6 Apply individual false lashes to the outer corner of upper eye if desired.

7 Choose a true red for the lipstick – the colours of the day were cherry, ruby, geranium, crimson, magenta, cerise and raspberry. Apply generously to the whole lip area.

8 Apply crème blusher to the apple of the cheeks.

EQUIPMENT AND PRODUCT LIST
Equipment and products for a 1930s make-up look
Equipment
Full make-up kit and brushes
Products
Eyebrow wax
Red lipstick
White eyeshadow

The 1940s

Due to World War II, 'normal life', including the progression of fashion, ceased. Therefore, there are many similarities between the make-up worn in the 1930s and that of the 1940s. However, the symbol of the era was lipstick, as that was the only item of make-up available during the war, although colours were limited, with red being the mainstay. Eyebrows were brushed neatly, kept in a natural shape and were usually darkened.

Main features of 1940s make-up

- Foundation   natural
- Eyebrows   brushed neatly, natural shape and darkened
- Eyes   natural
- Lips   red
- Cheeks   subtle shading
- Overall look   simple and sophisticated

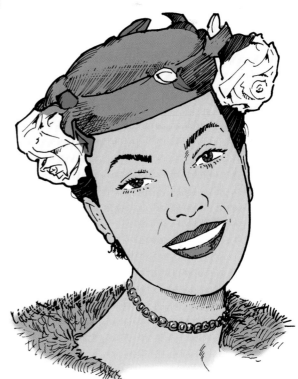

A fashionable lady of the 1940s

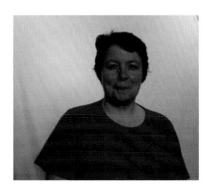

Early 1950s before

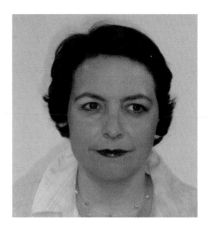

Early 1950s final

The 1950s

After the dark years of World War II, the 1950s saw an explosion of colour as Britain moved from the austerity of the 1940s to the prosperity of the 1950s. The coronation of Queen Elizabeth II took place in 1953 and millions of people in the UK and elsewhere in the world watched on small screen black and white television sets. This increased ownership of television sets also gave the population a chance to view the latest fashions in clothes and make-up. After the minimal look of 1940s make-up, the 1950s took off in style and bright clothes and make-up epitomised post-war optimism. There was a shortage of men (because of the losses of World War II), which encouraged women to look as beautiful as possible in the hope of 'catching' a husband. There was a boom in the luxury beauty industry, led by Elizabeth Arden and Helena Rubenstein, and Avon 'called' for the first time, introducing door to door cosmetics reps. With new labour saving devices becoming available, such as the vacuum cleaner, women had more time to pamper themselves. The late 1950s also brought us Dusty Springfield with her Beehive hairstyle and dark eye-make-up, which were copied throughout Britain – thanks again to television and the broadcasting of the first and only popular music programme of the day – Top of the Pops – which is still running today.

During the 1950s, a range of influences including film, television, magazines, and the rock music scene created a new market grouping called 'teenagers'. A sudden flurry of consumer goods denied to war-torn Europe were available and a consumer boom was actively encouraged. These single young people with cash from paid work soon had their own fashions, music, cafes, milk bars and, by the end of the decade, even their own transport in the form of fuelled scooters. Teenagers suddenly dominated style in clothes, hairstyles and make-up. A generation gap began to emerge between parents and their offspring. It seemed almost unholy at the time and was viewed as rebellious but, compared to later anti-fashion and anarchic movements, it was all rather innocent.

In the 1950s colour films made an enormous impact on cosmetics. The huge cinema screens illuminated the unblemished appearance of stars and caused the make-up artist Max Factor to invent an everyday version of the foundation he used called 'Pan Cake', originally founded in the 1930s. This was a make-up to gloss over skin imperfections. He also introduced a range of eye shadows and lipsticks. In the later 1950s a company called Gala introduced pale shimmering lipsticks that contained titanium. This was added to tone down the brightness of products and resulted in lips with a pale shimmering gleam. The idea was extended to create frosted nail varnishes of pink, silver and a host of other colours.

The key feature to obtaining a traditional 1950s look is the eyeliner flick. Matching both eyes can be tricky and you may need several attempts before they are aligned, so it is advisable to apply foundation after the eyeliner. There were no iridescent, frosted or pearlised products during the 1950s.

Main features of 1950s make-up

- Foundation   natural
- Eyebrows   dark and strong
- Eyes   black eyeliner with flick

- Cheeks   subtle shading
- Overall look   strong and chic

Re-creating a 1950s look

1 Apply a natural coloured base and set with loose translucent powder.

2 Darken the eyebrows by drawing a line on the top of the natural brow, then intensify the colour by pencilling in between the hairs.

3 Apply individual false lashes if required.

4 Starting from the inside corner of the eyelid, and using liquid eyeliner, create the flick by lining all along the top lashes and taking this line out 1cm and up at a 45° angle.

5 Apply pale green eye shadow on the lids, followed by brown to shadow the socket line and highlight below the brow.

6 Pencil the natural lip line with red, then fill them in using a brush.

EQUIPMENT AND PRODUCT LIST
Equipment and products for a 1950s make-up look
Equipment
Full make-up kit and brushes
Products
Black liquid eyeliner
Individual false eyelashes
Dark brown eyebrow pencil
Red lipstick

MAKE-UP THROUGH THE CENTURIES

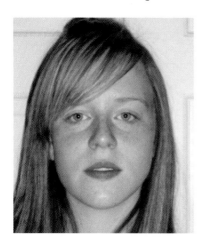

1950s before

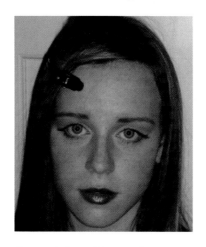

Stages 1, 2 and 3 – apply foundation and powder to set. Enhance eyebrows and fix false eyelashes

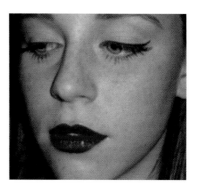

Stage 4 – apply eyeliner and flick to 45° angle

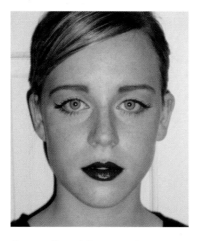

Stages 5 and 6 – complete eye make-up. Apply red lip liner and fill in using same colour

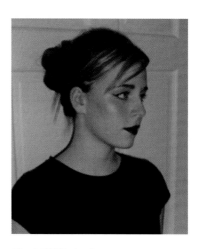

Final 1950s look

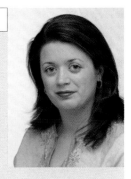

MAKE-UP ARTIST PROFILE: ADÉLE PALMER

How and when did you start in the business?

After finishing a fine art degree I was disappointed with the lack of opportunities for me so I wanted to find a creative career in something that really interested me. After some research I found a course in make-up for fashion and photography which I started in January 2004, and haven't looked back.

Was there a turning point in your career?

My first paid job. You can be the best in your class but when you get your first job it's such a good feeling to be paid to do something you really enjoy.

What do you consider to be important qualities for a make-up artist?

A soft touch … blend, blend, blend!!!! On a shoot you should be prepared with lots of ideas to discuss with the rest of the team but be confident enough to work independently. ALWAYS stick to the time scale given for the shoot.

What is your most memorable/exciting/best paid job?

Most memorable and best paid job has to be when I did the make-up for the guys who present 'Queer Eye for the Straight Guy', they were being interviewed on television and just HAD to have a make-up artist.

Have you had any disasters?

No disasters as such. Although on one shoot there was a lack of communication, I was asked for a Mexican/Brazilian look on the model. After I had spent nearly an hour doing gorgeous bronzed skin and smoky eyes I was then told that the look was 50s/Audrey Hepburn!!! Luckily we used sunglasses and I quickly changed to red lips!!

What advice would you give to young people entering the industry?

Find as many contacts as possible and keep in touch with them, you'll be surprised how many friends of friends know someone who can put a good word in for you. Be patient, it doesn't happen overnight.

In your experience, would you advise those training to become make-up artists to specialise in one area only, or to gain experience, through Continued Professional Development courses (CPD) in many different areas of make-up?

I would recommend finding one area you are strong in and really enjoy and specialise in that. Gain as much experience as possible; the best way to learn is to be out there with a professional seeing them work and finding out what's new.

The 1960s

In the early 1960s Max Factor brought out a colour called Strawberry Meringue which was a pastel pearly pink. These pearly pink lipsticks really caught on in the 1960s as young girls were frowned upon if they wore 'brazen' red lips. The softened pink and peach colours were initially acceptable to parents, but then became a trend. The eyes were the key feature of 1960s make-up, so a pale lip colour was used to enhance them. Magazines gave step-by-step instructions on how to use the recently introduced lip brushes and young girls began to blend and mix their own lip colours, often having first blotted the lips out with Max Factor Pancake make-up. Nail polish followed a similar trend, with pastel pearl colours being the rage. After the film Cleopatra was released, showing Elizabeth Taylor with very emphasised eyes, everyone learnt to apply eyeliner and socket lines. The models Jean Shrimpton and Twiggy (Leslie Hornby), along with the actress Julie Christie, with their lined eye sockets, captured the look that said 'Sixties Chick with chic'!

Mary Quant brought out a range of affordable cosmetics in 'up to the minute' formulations, with innovative cheek contour shaders and highlighters. She encouraged users to use make-up brushes to apply eyeliner and blusher to achieve the 'hollow cheek wide eyed' look of the model Twiggy. It really was the best make-up to use in that era if you wanted to get the right look, as it contained information leaflets with diagrams of positions for the blush shading and highlighting which was very innovative at the time. Many of the items she designed bore the Quant daisy logo, still used today.

Main features of 1960s make-up

- Foundation   pale
- Eyebrows   natural
- Eyes   smoky eye, false lashes, 'painted on' lower lashes
- Lips   pale pinks
- Cheeks   natural with a hint of colour over the apples of the cheeks
- Overall look   authenticate the look by adding typical black and white accessories, earrings, clothes, nails

Re-creating a 1960s look

1 Start with the eyeliner on the top lid. This should not be a thin eyeliner line, but a much wider line. Extend the natural line outwards by about $\frac{1}{2}$ cm (not an upward 1950s flick but just a natural extension of the eyelid line). This line can also extend into the inner corner of the eye, and even on to the side of the nose if the shape of the face and features allows.

2 Draw a similar line, this time over the socket line. Start with a black eyeliner pencil and, once you are satisfied with the shape, paint in with the black cake eyeliner. Once you are confident, you can apply the black cake eyeliner directly on the socket line.

3 Next you are going to draw in the lashes. Starting with the outer edge, use your extended line as a guide, and draw in about six lashes, starting with the longest and getting shorter as you move in towards the inner eye. Only draw in lashes for about half the length of the eye. Where the lashes meet the lid, draw in an additional dot, to accentuate the lashes.

4 Using white eyeliner, line the inner, lower rim of the eyes – this will open up the whole area (optional).

EQUIPMENT AND PRODUCT LIST

Equipment and products for a 1960s make-up look

Equipment

Full make-up kit and brushes

Products

Black cake eyeliner

Black eyeliner pencil

White eyeliner pencil

Black mascara

Concealer – for skin and lips

Eyelash curlers

5 Curl lashes, and apply black mascara liberally to both top and bottom lashes, leaving them cloggy for an authentic look.

6 The lips need to be neutral. Pat in either a concealer or a specialised lip product.

7 Use concealer around the nose, eyes, and anywhere else it is needed; apply pale foundation and complete the look with a little pink blusher to the apple of the cheek.

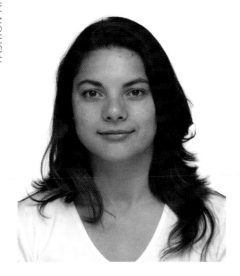

1960s before

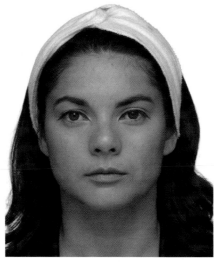

Stage 1 – apply eyeliner to top lid

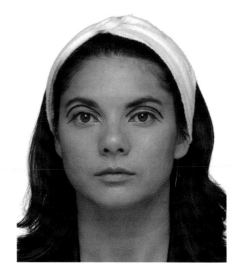

Draw a similar line over the socket line

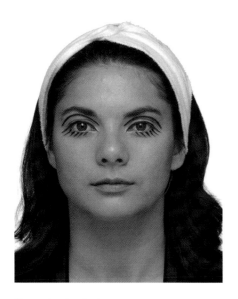

Draw in the lashes

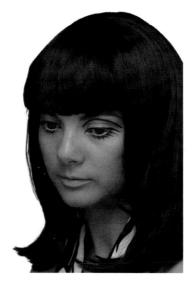

The completed look with white eyeliner to the lower rim of eyes, lashes curled, black mascara, and a little pink blusher

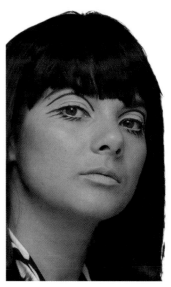

Updated 1960s look adding colour

Colour was not used in a traditional 1960s eye make-up. The last picture in this sequence shows how colour can update, or simply change a traditional look. This coloured version of a 1960s look would now suit a catwalk or pop video look.

MAKE-UP ARTIST PROFILE: SUE CALLAGHAN

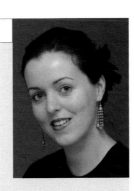

How and when did you start in the business?

I come from a fine art background but have always loved make-up. I did a course and started to get work whilst studying, after lots of networking.

Was there a turning point in your career?

I find that in this industry, things begin to snowball after your first job. It's definitely a confidence thing.

What do you consider to be important qualities for a make-up artist?

You must be able to get on with everyone and really make the effort to be friendly and useful. Being adaptable and open to new ideas at short notice, being able to work to a brief and of course creative talent.

What is your most memorable/exciting/best paid job?

Designing make-up for a new designer's fashion show, which was screened on the BBC, as I was able to work with designers and be very creative with ideas.

Have you had any disasters?

Not yet!

What advice would you give to young people entering the industry?

Go for it, you have to really believe in yourself. It is good to surround yourself with a support network, as in the beginning it is hard, as jobs can be few and far between. Also get as much experience as you can, as sometimes something you wouldn't expect to enjoy, you can really fall in love with.

In your experience, would you advise those training to become make-up artists to specialise in one area only, or to gain experience, through Continued Professional Development courses (CPD) in many different areas of make-up?

To start with I think a course where you learn about different areas is the best option as afterwards you begin to have preferences, which you can continue to develop, perhaps in one or two areas. The more you know the more chance you have of getting work and I think make-up is one of those things where you can never stop learning.

The 1970s

After a decade of distinctive dark smoky eyes and pale coloured lips during the 1960s, the 1970s brought a welcome change with big bold colour and iridescent powders.

Foundation was light, almost translucent and concealer used only where really necessary to conceal blemishes, or under the eyes where the skin becomes thinner. Concealer was not used right under the lashes because eye shadow was applied in this area.

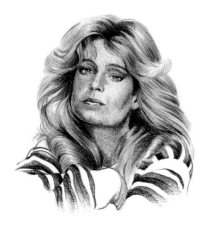

Farrah Fawcett

Unlike some other looks where a traditional foundation is used (foundation, concealer and powder), a 1970s look used no powder, leaving the skin slightly tacky, particularly in the eye area, in order for the iridescent powers to 'stick'. A little powder may have been used over the cheek area, when all the iridescent work was complete around the eyes.

Two colours were usually chosen for the eyes. One bright, dominant colour, such as a turquoise, or emerald green was used on the lower lid and taken under the lower lashes, and one pearly/white/silvery colour for the upper lid and under the brow. Both colours remained bold with just the hard edge being blended. There were no hard lines to be seen in 1970s make-up.

Softer browns replaced the harsh blacks of the 1960s. Brown pencil eyeliner was applied to the inner rim of the bottom lid and brown mascara applied to top and bottom lashes. A 'cloggy' mascara was all part of the 1970s look.

Blusher was applied to under the cheekbones, and lips were coloured with pale lipstick, as the main emphasis was the eyes.

To complete the look, iridescent powder was used under the brow area, in the corners of the eyes, above the cheekbones and over the cupid's bow, to emphasise the shapes of these areas.

Main features of 1970s make-up

- Foundation   light
- Eyebrows   high and arched
- Eyes   two colours – one bright, the other pearly
- Lips   pale and pearly
- Cheeks   blusher applied under the cheekbones and highlighter on the cheekbones
- Overall look   glitzy

EQUIPMENT AND PRODUCT LIST

Equipment and products for a 1970s make-up look

Equipment

Full make-up kit and brushes

Products

Glitters and iridescent powders

Pearly lipsticks

White eyeliner

Re-creating a 1970s look

1 Choose the products to be used – have everything ready before you start.

2 Cleanse, tone and moisturise the face.

3 Apply foundation to the face – don't rush: remember that the foundation is the most important part of any make-up.

4 Starting with the eyes, apply the dominant eye colour to the lower lids, and the second colour, the pearly/white/silvery colour to the upper lid. Blend the hard lines together.

5 Take the lower lid colour and apply under the lashes, not as an eyeliner but as a deeper line of colour, right over to the inner edge of the eye.

6 Using a brown eyeliner, line the inside rims of the eyes.

7 Using brown mascara, apply to top and bottom lashes – don't worry if the mascara clogs, it is all part of the 1970s look.

8 Apply blusher to under the cheek bones.

9   Choosing a light, not too dominant colour, fill in the lips using a lip brush.

10 Check all foundation is still in place, and correct if it is not.

11 Lightly apply a translucent powder.

12 Taking an iridescent powder, apply sparingly to just below the brow, to the inside of the eye, over the cheekbones and to the cupid's bow, to highlight these areas.

TIP

Iridescent powders and anything with glitter or sparkle should be kept in a separate bag from your other make-up. Glitters get everywhere – keep everything else covered when you are using it, as there is nothing worse than if you get some sparkle or glitter on a straight make-up. This is true of brushes too – keep a separate set of brushes for sparkle/glitter work in the same box as the products – you will be glad you did!

The early 1970s saw a 1920s revival in the use of doll-like features. The make-up company Biba hit on this for an advertising campaign. The Biba look is illustrated here.

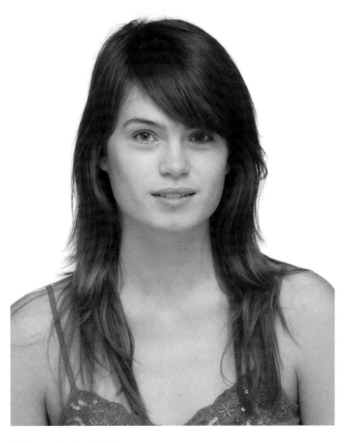

Before photo 1970s

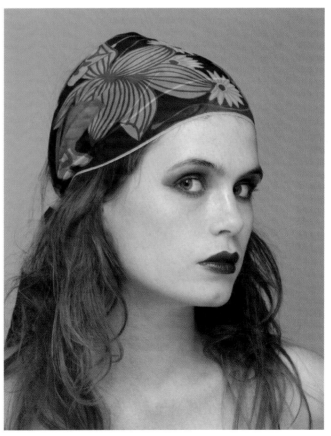

Completed 'Biba' look

MAKE-UP ARTIST PROFILE: TAMSIN PYNE

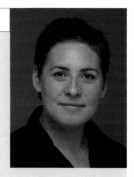

How and when did you start in the business?

Aged 27, I found myself at a 'career junction' having graduated with a business studies degree and trained as an English Language teacher but still not professionally fulfilled. I loved make-up from a very early age and in later years had done the make-up for quite a few weddings whilst still working in an office full time.

I decided to train formally in January 2004 and chose a very reputable school in London to study Fashion & Photographic Make-up.

Was there a turning point in your career?

My career is still in its infancy, though taking the leap to change career completely was a big turning point in my life.

What do you consider to be important qualities for a make-up artist?

I believe a good make-up artist can be separated from the rest if they have an eye for detail, patience, artistic flair and good team work ethics.

What is your most memorable/exciting/best paid job?

The most memorable and exciting was my first job. It involved pizza, chocolate muffins and heaps of laughter! It was a poster/billboard shoot advertising a company of comedians who were performing at Edinburgh's Fringe Festival 2004. The photographer had an amazing portfolio of portraits of famous comedians, so I was a little nervous! But he was such fun and totally chilled out. The comedians had to get into character for their photos so the make-up had to reflect this, thus testing my interpreting skills. The shoot took three full days, so we all got to know each other, ordered in pizza and muffins, and I have stayed in touch with some of the team.

Have you had any disasters?

Not on any professional jobs, but on friends whilst experimenting with new make-up, yes!!!

What advice would you give to young people entering the industry?

Be prepared for periods without work whilst you build your portfolio and reputation. Don't close any doors, you never know where they may lead. There are lots of good websites that advertise work so get on the net.

In your experience, would you advise those training to become make-up artists to specialise in one area only, or to gain experience, through Continued Professional Development courses (CPD) in many different areas of make-up?

I trained in a very specific field first because, at the time, I was totally sure of the direction I wanted my career to take. But subsequently and in the future I would like to gain wider experience. So it's probably best to have a broader knowledge before you specialise.

The 1980s

Bold matt colours replaced the iridescents of the 1970s. The 1980s saw a decade of power dressing which inspired striking make-up with deep pigments in all colours. Celebrities like Joan Collins, Jerry Hall and Cindy Crawford epitomised this look, setting the trend for the general public.

Main features of 1980s make-up

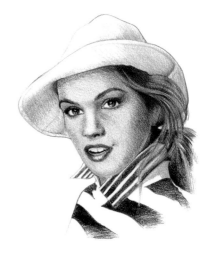

Cindy Crawford

- Foundation   natural foundation
- Eyebrows   natural
- Eyes   colourful socket lining
- Lips   strong colours
- Cheeks   heavy use of blusher under or on the cheekbones
- Overall look   bold, strong and brash!

The 1990s

The 1990s was a decade of individualism. Looks from past eras started creeping back into fashion and were adopted by the younger generation, whilst the majority of women knew what suited them in fashion and make-up and stayed with their adopted style. The damage the sun caused to skin became fully appreciated in the 1990s and an explosion of self-tanning creams and bronzers hit the market. Cosmetics were more about skin care and anti-ageing products than make-up. The main features are difficult to define, as there were so many different styles throughout the decade. The majority of women chose a natural look make-up – well applied.

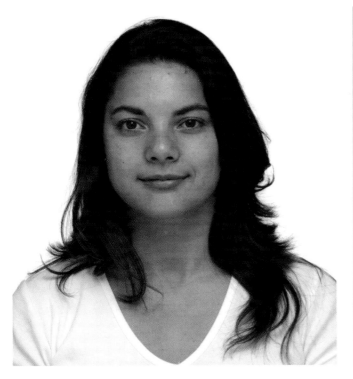

1990s before

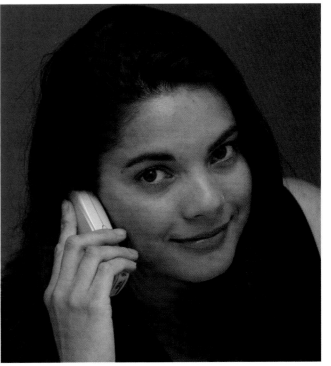

The natural look of the 1990s

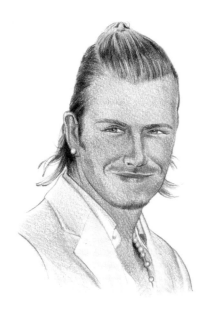

David Beckham in earrings

Present trends

Present trends are very individual. Women still know what suits them and they tend to stick with a look they are comfortable with. Younger women are veering towards the 1950s fashions again – not only in make-up, introducing the 1950s 'flick' into the twenty-first century, but with flared skirts and pointed shoes. There are still fringe groups – as there always will be – 'Goths' for example, where anything goes, so long as it is black: eyes, lips, nails and clothes. Temporary and permanent tattoos were also popular at the beginning of the twenty-first century, see Chapter 13, 'Face and Body Painting'.

Futuristic

Who knows what trends there will be in the future? Celebrities still have the ability to set trends. David Beckham, for example, set a trend when he began to wear diamond earrings. Many men up to that point had worn a single stud or hoop, but now that David was wearing a 'pair' of earrings, it became acceptable for other men to follow. David Beckham also started wearing pink nail varnish – that didn't become as trendy as the earrings, but who knows what may have happened since the time of writing? If men in the eighteenth century wore wigs and frilly shirts, why shouldn't twenty-first century man wear make-up and jewellery?

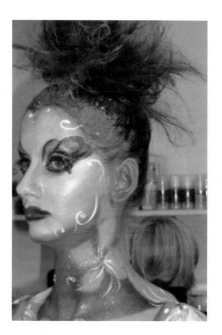

Futuristic head and neck

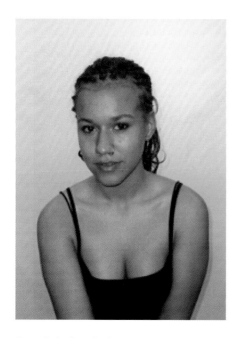

Futuristic face before

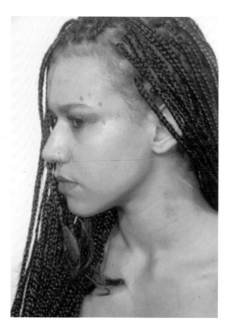

Futuristic face stage 1

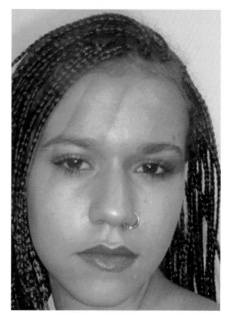

Futuristic face final look

STRAIGHTFORWARD MALE MAKE-UP

EQUIPMENT AND PRODUCT LIST

Equipment and products for a straightforward male make-up

Equipment

Full make-up kit and brushes

Products

Clear mascara

Vaseline

Men will often have facial hair or stubble and care must be taken not to get any foundation on it.

1 Cleanse, tone and moisturise the skin, removing excess moisturiser by blotting the skin with a tissue.

2 Apply foundation to the face using a sponge, starting at the centre and working outwards so that you do not clog the hairline with make-up. Do not take foundation up to the eye; blend into this area instead, otherwise it makes the make-up too obvious. Once the foundation is blended, any blemishes that need to be concealed can be covered using a concealer. Do this with a dabbing motion with either your fingertip or a small brush. Our model has a scar above his left eyebrow, so by applying a concealer in a lighter tone than his skin colour in the recess of the scar, and in one shade darker around the outside of the scar, this has the effect of 'lifting' the scar and making the skin look level.

3 Powder the face – it is important not to use too much powder when working on men, as they will look 'made-up'.

4 Brush the eyebrows through to remove any make-up residue. In our example, the eyebrow with the scar was filled-in using an eyebrow pencil to cover where the hair does not grow.

5 Apply a very light dusting of blusher to the cheeks and finally wipe the lips with a clean sponge – to remove any foundation.

6 Apply a very small amount of Vaseline – to give a healthier appearance.

7 To remove – cleanse, tone and moisturise.

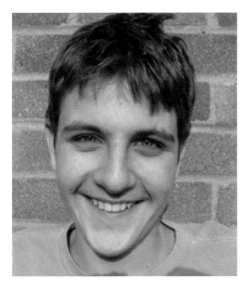

Before look for male make-up

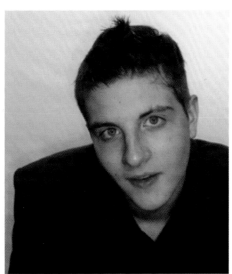

After look for male make-up

FASHION LOOKS FOR EDITORIAL WORK AND FASHION SHOWS

Editorial work

Editorial work generally involves close-up portrait work where very precise make-up is needed. The illustrations here show examples of editorial work that covers many different make-up styles. Practise these looks, they are not as easy as they look! The 'fresh and freckles' look is a complete make-up, although it may appear as if there is no make-up at all – that is the art of fashion make-up. Practise pastel looks as well to get variations in your portfolio.

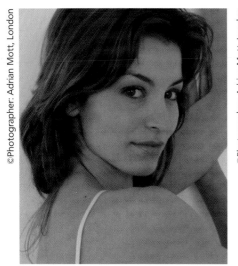

©Photographer: Adrian Mott, London

Editorial – natural make-up

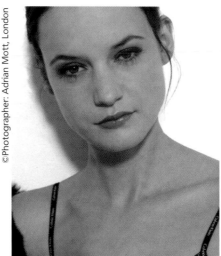

©Photographer: Adrian Mott, London

Editorial – soft and subtle

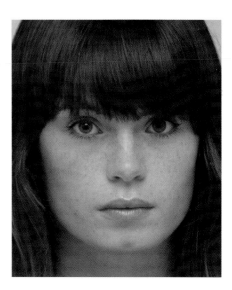

Editorial Fresh and freckles

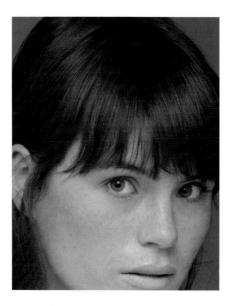

Editorial – pastels

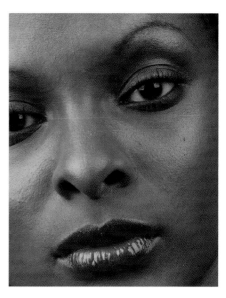

Editorial – Black by Design Make-up

Quite often a magazine will run a 'story book' feature, where the make-up on a model is adapted several times to produce different, but related looks. In the series of pictures shown here, the common feature in each look is the lemon yellow eye shadow colour. Look 1 is for the daytime and is fresh and natural. Look 2 has been intensified with a darker shade of lipstick and for the final look eyeliner, mascara and an even darker shade of lipstick have been applied to create a romantic night time look.

STUDENT ACTIVITY

8.3   Search through some magazines for story book features.

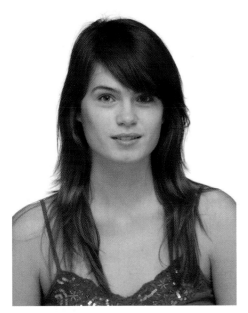

Story book – before

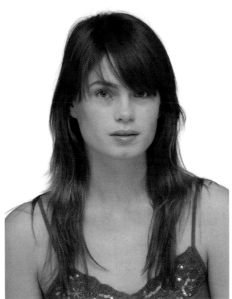

Story book – look 1

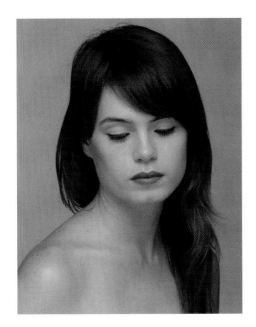

Story book – look 2 – intensified colour and lip colour introduced

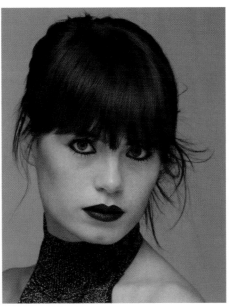

Story book – look 3 – darker again for a romantic evening look

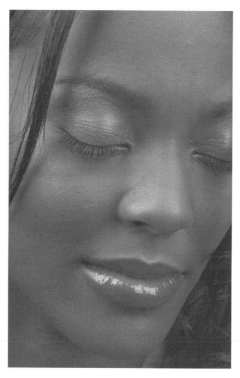

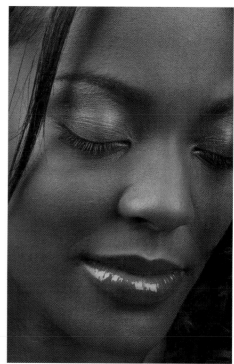

Editorial – Black by Design Make-up   Editorial – Black by Design Make-up

Always consider what your work will look like if printed as a black and white print instead of a colour print.

Fashion shows, catwalks and pop videos

These events frequently call for very creative, cutting edge looks.

However, in the Prada looks of 2002 and 2003, it appeared as if no colour had been used at all – just foundation and shine over the temples. However, shading and highlighting were clearly used instead.

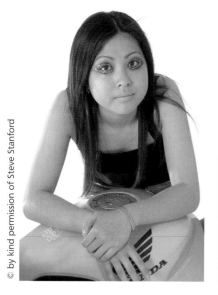

Catwalk – pop video look

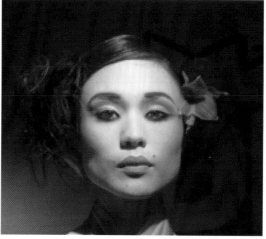

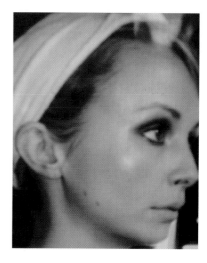

Catwalk – dramatic use of colour   Catwalk – the Prada look

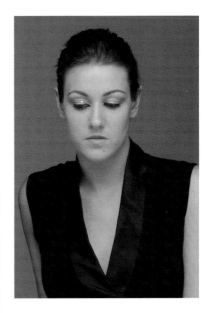

Fashion show – using glitters

Although some very dramatic make-up has been seen on catwalks, there is often an adopted style that is varied for each model within a show. For example, glitter may be used, in the same style but with different colours.

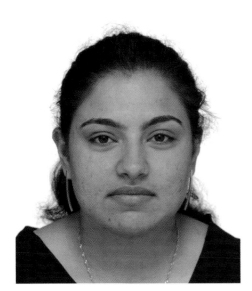

Fashion show – before

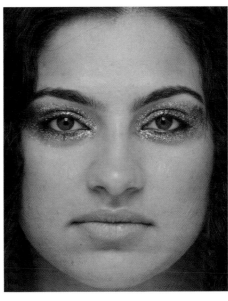

Fashion show – using purple glitter

Long eye make-up

This is an interesting eye look and one that is often used in magazine and fashion looks. It is particularly suitable for close set eyes, as the extended outer edge 'extends' the eye, making it look longer.

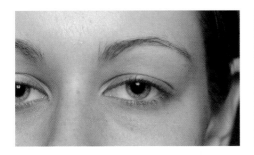

Long eye before

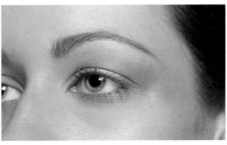

Long eye final

Smoky eye look

The smoky eye look can be quite dramatic and is often used for catwalk/fashion show make-up. Look through fashion magazines and you will find many examples of the smoky eye look. Brown is its traditional colour, but you can also use grey/black, royal blue or dark greens. The emphasis of this look is that it is very dark and very blended. It resembles a 'bull's eye' – dark in the centre and getting lighter and lighter as the circle moves out – the hard edge needs to be blended well.

When applying eye make-up for fashion and photography, it must be symmetrical. Stand immediately in front of your model when applying the make-up, and. from time to time, stand behind the model and look at their reflection in a mirror, if this is possible. What may look perfect close up, may not look as perfect from a distance, as peoples' faces are not symmetrical. Always keep in mind the end result, be it a photograph for a magazine, or a model on a catwalk.

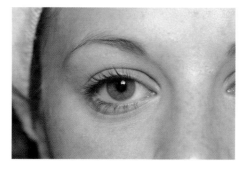

Catwalk before

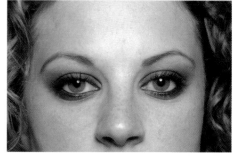

Catwalk – smoky eye look

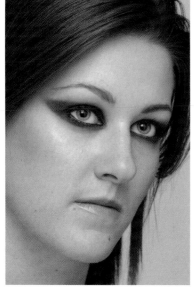

Fashion show – cats eye

Cat eye

As you can see from the photo, this is a very dramatic look, which drags the eyes upward like a cat. It is often used in fashion shows on the catwalk!

Strong eye shadow and pigments

When working in fashion settings, you can explore your own creativity to the full. Bright colours dominate – and there are no right or wrong techniques to follow. What is important is a dramatic end result.

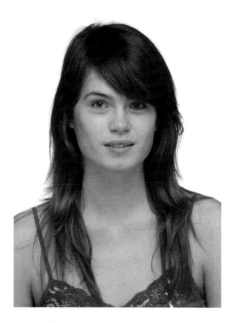

Catwalk – strong eye and brow shadows and pigments before

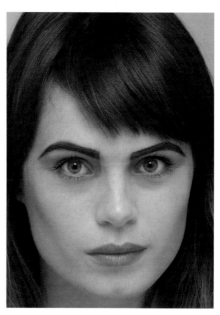

Catwalk – strong eye and brow shadows and pigments final

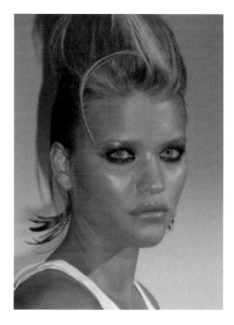

Catwalk – smoky eye

Catalogues

The emphasis in this situation is on the clothes; the make-up is not quite as cutting edge as for fashion shows. Its market is more the general public rather than fashion critics and buyers. Catalogues tend to be looking for natural, beautiful make-up.

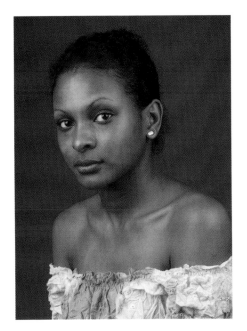

Catalogue – Black by Design make-up

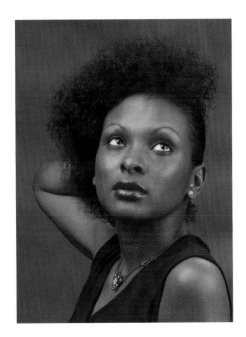

Catalogue – Black by Design make-up

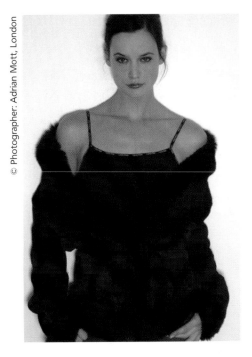

© Photographer: Adrian Mott, London

Catalogue – editorial from page 124 becomes catalogue, showing off the clothes as well as the make-up

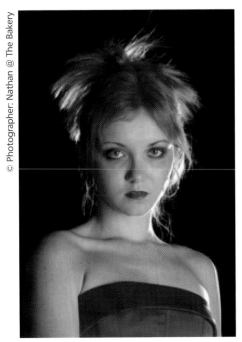

© Photographer: Nathan @ The Bakery

Catalogue – a typical catalogue image

Assessment of knowledge and understanding

Knowledge review

1 What factor should you consider when choosing lipstick (or the colour of any make-up) for a black and white photograph?

2 Why does photographic/beauty work need to be perfect?

3 Why is learning the make-up fashions of past eras important?

4 What particular feature of the seventeenth-century make-up was used to cover skin imperfections?

5 What was the general shape of lips in the eighteenth century?

6 What were Queen Victoria's views on make-up?

7 What made women of the 1920s so different?

8 What are the main features of a 1920s make-up?

9 What are the main features of a 1930s make-up?

10 What are the two most apparent features of a 1950s make-up?

11 What are the main features of a 1960s make-up?

12 What was different about 1970s make-up?

13 How can a Biba look be described?

14 What does editorial work involve?

15 What is a story book feature?

16 How are fashion shows/catwalks and pop video make-up described?

17 How can you describe the 2002 and 2003 Prada look?

18 Why is the long eye look suitable for magazines and fashion looks?

19 What is the emphasis of the smoky eye look?

20 What is the make-up emphasis of catalogue work?

chapter 9

Planning and promoting make-up activities

The aims of planning and promoting make-up activities in beauty salons and cosmetic houses are to promote the business and increase business revenue. The planning and promoting of make-up activities include offering individual make-up lessons, group demonstrations and fashion shows. The intention of these activities is to increase consumer awareness of products and to sell stock. Therefore, included in the planning and promoting of make-up activities is selling techniques and stock control – very important aspects of working in a beauty salon or cosmetic house.

Learning objectives

In this chapter you will learn about:

- **make-up lessons**
- **group make-up demonstrations**
- **fashion shows**
- **stock control**
- **selling cosmetics**

THE MAKE-UP LESSON

A popular beauty salon and cosmetic house service is the make-up lesson. You will encounter a wide range of clients: young women who are looking for the correct way to apply make-up, middle-aged ladies who want to change the look of their make-up, older ladies who may never have worn much make-up but who now feel they need some to conceal emerging lines and wrinkles. You may even encounter male models who are seeking instruction in the application of make-up either for personal use, for a theatrical production or for a fancy dress party. Be prepared for all kinds of requests!

The main difference between a beauty salon make-up service and a cosmetics make-up service is that in the beauty salon the client will apply the make-up herself, whereas in a cosmetics store the make-up artist will apply all the products. The beauty salon is a much more relaxed, personal and private service. In a cosmetics store, the lesson can often be rushed, impersonal and very public.

A competent therapist/make-up artist needs patience and good communication skills as the instructions she gives need to be clear. Start with a full consultation and include the following questions:

1 For what particular reason is the client having this make-up lesson?
2 What are his/her expectations of the lesson?
3 Is he/she prepared to purchase new products to acquire the new look?

There are a couple of ways to instruct a client who has come for a make-up lesson. You can either give guidance and instruction and let the client do all the application herself – which can take a long time – or you can apply half the face and let the client complete the other half. Ask the client which approach she would like you to take. We will assume the second approach has been chosen for our example make-up lesson: the make-up artist will apply half the make-up and the client will apply the other half.

Ask the client's permission to take two 'before' photographs of the usual make-up style. A Polaroid camera is excellent for this. Often, clients cannot remember the 'before' look once the new look has been established. Once the make-up is complete, take another two photos – again with permission. Give one set of these photographs to the client to show to family and friends, to act as a reminder of the two looks and to get feedback. (Sometimes clients will have the make-up removed before leaving the salon.) The other set of photos is for your portfolio of evidence.

An individual make-up lesson

Allocated time: $1^1/_2$–2 hours

A client will be slower to apply make-up than you. She will be learning new techniques, using new products and maybe using brushes for the first time, so allowing sufficient time is really important, especially as you want to recommend retail items to her at the end of the lesson.

Our example shows a client who has worn heavy eye make-up for the past 30 years – since the 1960s in fact! She is now a grandmother, albeit a young one, and requires a softer more mature look. The make-up lesson can take any order of application you feel appropriate.

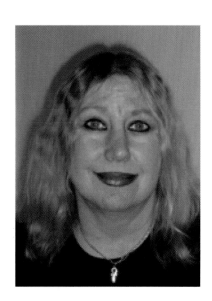

1 Start with a full consultation to establish your client's personal details, face shape and other features. As you decide on the colours and products to be used, you should complete a make-up worksheet. This will act as an aide memoire for you and your client of the colours you have actually used.

2 Tie the client's hair back with a hair band before you start. You will need to cleanse, tone and moisturise the skin before any application of make-up and it is strongly recommended that the therapist/make-up artist do this to save valuable time.

3 You can sit next to each other, either alongside a therapy couch or at a worktop. Wherever you sit, the client needs to have full use of a mirror. Aim for natural light so the client can see the true colours you have both chosen and she will be using. The client needs to apply the make-up herself, as this is what she has come to you to learn. You should demonstrate as necessary, but then let her try as well. Do not be tempted to do it for her! A total make-up application by the therapist/make-up artist is another service entirely.

4 Having completed the consultation sheet and decided upon a new realistic and achievable make-up look for the client, take out the product choices and decide on the colours to be used. All products are chosen first, as this also saves a lot of valuable time when you eventually start to apply the make-up. Demonstrate to her how to choose a perfect foundation colour to match her skin tone. Test the foundation at the jaw line and the colour that appears to disappear is the correct colour. Don't forget to take undertones into account. Having chosen a foundation colour, a concealing product is chosen in the same colour. Then proceed to choose all the colours you need for the look you are going to make.

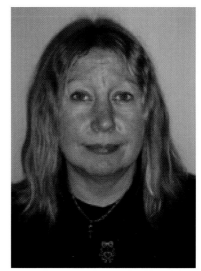

TIP

1$\frac{1}{2}$–2 hours will elapse very quickly. Choosing all the colours before you start the make-up application will save you valuable time.

5 Having selected appropriate colours, put all other make-up away. Display the chosen products in their order of use. Explain the importance of using make-up brushes to get a good finish. Lay out the brushes to be used and direct the client each time a change of brush is needed, explaining the function of each brush.

TIP

Encourage the client frequently – tell her she is doing well. Keep the session fun as well as professional.

6 You can now start with the application of the concealer and foundation. Using the correct brush, show her how to conceal any blemishes. Let her complete the second half of her face. Do the same with the foundation, using either a brush or a latex sponge wedge. It is probably not wise to set the make-up with powder at this stage. The client will almost undoubtedly drop eye shadow down onto the cheeks, which may make a mess and you don't want to have to start again. Complete the make-up and then set with powder.

7 Eyes – refer to your now completed make-up worksheet for the chosen style and make-up colours and products to be used, and proceed to make-up one eye. Talk through your movements with the client and let her study what you have done before she has a go herself.

TIP ✔

Don't do too much work on one eye at once. Smaller, 'bite sized' applications will be quicker in the long run.

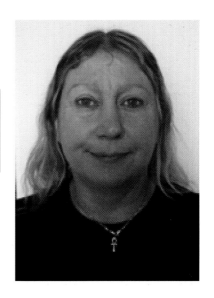

8 Complete the eyes using eyeliner and mascara following the same procedure.

9 Move onto the lips. Again following the same procedure, complete half the lips using a lip liner the same colour as the lip colour the client has chosen. The client will then complete the other half of her lips, before

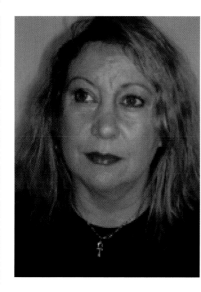

you fill in the lip area with the chosen colour and the client completes the procedure.

10 Proceed to shading and highlighting according to face shape, and set the make-up with powder if appropriate.

11 Remove hair band and arrange hair.

12 Take the 'after' photographs.

13 Always leave enough time at the end of the treatment to discuss the products that have been used with a view to selling them.

TIP

To maximise your profit from the appointment time, a product (or two) could be 'given' to the client as part of the service – the cost of which you will have included in the price of the treatment anyway. With 'free' products in her hand, she will be tempted to buy other products.

GROUP DEMONSTRATIONS

A group demonstration requires a little more planning than an individual lesson. The most important aspect of a group demonstration is not to make it too large. Everyone needs to be able to see what is going on! Seasonal demonstrations promoting the new season's products are always successful. Here is a checklist of points to take into consideration when planning an event of this nature.

- *Invitations* – if you send out invitations, the recipient immediately feels special and is more likely to attend than in response to an advertisement in the local paper. Send out invitations well in advance and include an RSVP (request to reply). You need to know exactly how many people are coming to the event in order for it to run smoothly. If you only run four group demonstrations a year, with limited numbers, clients will soon be asking to come – because you have made it exclusive.

- *Existing clients* – inviting existing clients to product demonstrations is a way to say thank you to them for being a regular client. However, you also want to attract new clients. Inviting an existing client with an 'introduce a friend' offer also works well.

- *Demonstration* – decide well in advance exactly what the demonstration will be, who will be demonstrating and on whom. Usually one member of staff making up another is a good idea. Practise the demonstration at least a couple of times before the event. You may decide to concentrate your demonstration on one particular product, or have a 'lips' promotion or a 'foundations' promotion, or you may decide to do a whole look. Demonstrating on somebody from the audience is not recommended. Don't let the demonstration be too long – 20–30 minutes is ideal.

- *Welcome* – have a good welcome ready for your guests. Offer plenty of cool drinks in the summer and warm drinks in the winter. Delegate a member of staff to looking after coats, and allow others to mingle with the guests.

- *Staff* – make sure there are enough staff working to look after the clients. The higher the ratio of staff to clients, the more successful the event will be. Don't forget to offer staff an incentive for working what will probably be outside their normal hours. Staff should all wear name tags, or distinctive clothing, so guests know who the staff are.

- *Timing* – early evenings are a good time. It is always advisable to hold demonstration events when the actual salon is closed. This also makes clients feel special. In addition, it allows you to give all your time to your guests and not be doing day to day business.

- *'Goodie bags'* – have 'goodie bags' for everyone to take home with them. Make sure your salon brochure is in the bag and any other promotional material that is relevant to the event. Let your suppliers know what you are doing. They will be only too pleased to supply you with free samples for the 'goodie bags'. You may want to include a discount card to be used before a certain date. Use the bags to your advantage.

- *Stock* – it is almost inevitable that guests will want to buy products at the end of the evening. The whole point of the event is to promote and sell a certain range or product, so you must ensure you have sufficient stock. Order this well in advance. You do not want the whole event spoiled because you didn't order in sufficient time. Tell your suppliers that you are holding an event to promote their product and they will probably send you posters and free stock to use on the night.

- *Start on time* – while it is very pleasant for your guests to mingle and network before your demonstration begins, it is important that you start promptly. The main business of the event – that of selling products – cannot begin until the demonstration is over.

- *Fun* – group demonstrations and events can be great fun and be very motivating for staff and clients alike.

- *Not just for the ladies* – men also like to go to events. Have a male event about six weeks before Christmas or a few weeks before St. Valentine's day, promoting presents for their loved ones or a new men's range of cosmetics.

FASHION SHOWS

Fashion shows need a lot of organising. If you are doing the make-up for a fashion show, it is imperative that you go to all the planning meetings. You need to know everything about the event. Often one or two ladies fashion outlets will get together with one beauty salon and put on a double promotion. Make sure, if you are the beauty salon or the make-up artist, that you get your fair share of the exposure. You will need to know the following well in advance:

- How many models there will be.
- Will there be a hairdresser?
- What type of clothes are being shown?
- How many changes of outfit are planned?
- What age group – models and audience.

- The location of the show.
- How many people are expected to be in the audience?
- Will there be space for a trade table at the show?
- Will there be an opportunity for you to hand out your own promotional material?
- Will there be posters advertising the event? If so, make sure your company name is big enough for all to see.
- Will there be any TV coverage? Again you want coverage too.

Being the make-up artist for a fashion show can be great fun and you can usually be very creative with your ideas, but the clothes do get the limelight. Make absolutely sure it is worth your while doing before committing yourself.

If the event is a small scale fashion show, you may be able to do a make-up demonstration in the interval. With video cameras and head microphones, a make-up demonstration in between the fashion can be fun. The most important thing to remember if you are taking part in a joint venture with any other company, is that you get your 50 per cent of the publicity.

STOCK CONTROL

Every retail establishment has its own methods for handling and controlling retail stock, which is a very important aspect of any business. You need enough stock on the shelves to be able to make a good display but you don't need so much that it affects the company's cash flow. Products can be expensive and many companies have minimum orders, so it is important that you re-order only what you really want and only items that you know you can sell. If your order does not meet the minimum order amount required by your supplier, consider changing supplier. With minimum orders, you are being forced to buy stock you do not really want – and no business can afford that. All successful businesses need to know who their customers are and what they want to buy.

HEALTH AND SAFETY

Do not leave old packing materials unattended – remove and dispose of promptly and correctly, according to establishment rules.

Receiving and processing the stock

This includes checking the stock against a delivery note. Often, items missing from delivered stock will not be replaced by the supplier. It is therefore important when signing for stock that you add to your signature 'unexamined' on the docket. Stock must be received, unpacked and stored according to the establishment rules on stock delivery.

Rotating stock

When new stock arrives, it must be placed behind the old stock, so that the old stock is sold first. Having to take unsold stock off shelves because it has not been sold, or because new stock has been sold first, or because it may have passed its 'best before' date is a gross mismanagement of company funds. New stock should be stored correctly, and the whole process of stock delivery should be carried out safely, hygienically and with minimum inconvenience to customers, clients and staff.

Recording and labelling stock

Stock is often kept in two places in many establishments. The majority of it is kept in a stock cupboard, and the remainder on the shelves and in display cabinets. As stock is moved from the cupboards to the display areas, all the necessary documentation must be completed according to establishment rules, to enable the person who re-orders to have up to date records of stock held. Stock in the stock cupboard should be stored in such a way that it can be seen and counted easily. Often there are divisions of stock – some for retail selling and some for use within the business. If this is the case, then the two different types of stock must be kept separate.

Displaying stock

Buying in stock is one thing, but unless it is displayed attractively, it may not sell. Display equipment is available either as free standing or fixed units and it can be difficult to estimate the amount of stock required to make a good display in the available space. Be artistic in your stock display. Do not overcrowd an area, but have enough stock so that clients are aware that it is for sale. Take care not to display perishable goods in the sunlight. A golden rule in stock display is to change it regularly. If you keep the same display for months on end, clients stop looking. But with standard displays, where stock can be found easily, and promotional displays that are different each month, clients will be kept interested.

> **HEALTH AND SAFETY**
>
> Any faulty display fixtures or equipment must be reported to management promptly. Display areas must be clean and tidy and free from hazards after construction.

SELLING COSMETICS

Selling cosmetics is often in the job description of beauty therapists and is an important part of the work. If you work in a cosmetics outlet, then selling cosmetics is the major part of the position. Here are some tips on good selling techniques:

- Be aware of the client's objectives in purchasing cosmetics. Identify your client's needs by using good listening and questioning skills. Practise using 'open' questions.
- Ask the client if she is intolerant to any cosmetic items or has any medically identified allergies – this will show her you care and she will be more likely to buy from you.
- Know the product – its functions, features and benefits. Learn the ingredients of any product you are selling – the customers will want to know what they are putting on their skin. If you don't know the answers, customers may walk away.
- Direct the client to the most suitable cosmetics to meet the identified objectives of their purchase. It is much easier recommending something a client actually needs than something they don't.
- Answer all questions, fully, clearly and accurately – you will be asked many.
- Possible contra-actions must be clearly explained.
- Never underestimate a customer's spending power.
- Maintain a professional manner at all times and be sensitive, supportive and respectful.

> **TIP**
>
> Open questions are questions that require a full answer; closed questions merely need a 'yes' or 'no' answer. Open-ended questions start with What, When, Which and Where. For example: 'What is your favourite colour lipstick?' would have a reply which is a colour – which opens up the conversation. On the other hand, 'Are you looking to buy any cosmetics today?' may result in a 'no' response, and the conversation is closed.

Assessment of knowledge and understanding

Knowledge review

1 What are the main aims of planning and promoting make-up activities?

2 What is the main difference between a beauty salon make-up service and a cosmetics store make-up service?

3 What are the two ways to instruct a client who has come for a make-up lesson?

4 Why should you take a photograph of the model before the make-up lesson?

5 For what reason should you allow sufficient time at the end of the make-up lesson?

6 What health and safety aspect should you consider when unpacking stock?

7 What are the advantages of sending out invitations for group demonstrations?

8 What are the advantages of holding a demonstration out of hours?

9 Why should you ensure that you have sufficient stock at a group demonstration?

10 Name six items of information you need to know in advance of a fashion show.

chapter 10

Wigs and postiche

Make-up artists are often required to provide wigs and postiche for media make-up as part of normal workplace procedures. Although you will not have to make wigs yourself, you do need to be able to measure for and apply wigs and hairpieces. It is also useful to be able to identify different types of wigs and postiche and to understand the wigmaking process. This will help you when commissioning or hiring wigs and with your communication skills when you talk with other people about the subject. Wigs are often used to create historical and period looks and to change the appearance of a character, but can also be required due to an illness and/or disease that may have caused baldness. The hairpiece can be as small as a false eyelash or as large as a wig. Postiche work for the face includes beards, moustaches, sideburns and eyebrows.

Learning objectives

In this chapter you will learn about:

- **wigs**
  - **consultation procedures**
  - **how to measure a model for a wig**
  - **different types of wigs and hairpieces**
  - **how to set a wig or hairpiece**
  - **how to apply a wig or hairpiece**

- **postiche work – facial hair**
  - **applying facial hair directly to the skin**
  - **different types of hair used in theatrical make-up**
  - **preparing, combing, mixing and applying crepe hair**
  - **stubble**
  - **female to male make-up**

- **applying false lashes – strip and individual**

WIGS

Wigs are used for numerous reasons:

- for historical and period looks
- to change the sex of a model
- to change the character of a model
- to make a model look older or younger
- to create a fantasy or an illusion
- to make a model more glamorous
- to represent authority, for example legal wigs
- for people who have lost their own hair through illness
- to achieve an illusion of baldness (bald wigs)

Different types of wigs and hairpieces

'Weft' work is the weaving of hair in the manufacture of postiche. The hair is interwoven onto silks, cotton thread or wire – interweaving at the root ends forms lengths of weft. The weft is folded, spirally wound, or sewn onto a mount or base. Wigs made in this way are known as weft wigs and many other pieces of postiche use woven or weft work. Weft work is useful for adding to natural hair to provide extra bulk and length in period hair work.

Simple weft wig

Simple weft wigs are mass-produced synthetic fibres or reduced hair wigs that are made in various sizes. The foundation is made of machine-sewn vegetable net. Wigs made from synthetic fibres cannot be styled or changed whilst those made from hair that has been reduced by acids can be styled with limitations. Simple weft wigs are often used on stage or screen, and are ideal for crowd scenes.

Hand-knotted wigs

Hand-knotted pieces and wigs are more expensive than mass-produced wigs, although the quality of the finish may not be suitable for TV and film.

Consultation procedures

Before measuring for a wig or hairpiece, it is necessary to establish the model's exact requirements and expectations. First, you will need all the usual information such as their name and address, age and contact numbers. At this point, give each client a unique reference number. You need to know the purpose of the wig – a theatre or media production or private use. You will then have to establish the style, length, density, colour and texture required (especially if the client has already lost all their hair), and whether the hair is to be curly or straight.

Measuring the model for a wig

For a wig to fit correctly, the head must be measured in a number of different dimensions and the measurements recorded. The head is covered and a template made which can be sent to a wigmaker. The order for the wig must meet a plan approved by the client. The need for accuracy cannot be stressed enough – if measurements are not taken accurately, valuable time and money may be lost.

Why is measuring important? Have you ever seen people whose toupees, wigs or hairpieces are slipping off? Or did a difference in colour from that natural hair draw your attention to it? These people probably bought their pieces 'off the shelf' and consequently they did not fit properly and were the wrong colour match. If accurate measurements are taken, the wigmaker has the necessary information to make a postiche that not only fits *perfectly*, but is also a perfect colour match. Sending a photograph of the client to the wigmaker with the order is very helpful, so that he/she may see the client's features. Face shape, hairline and visible abnormalities like cysts or bumps, whether the client wears glasses or a hearing aid are all aspects that may affect the finished piece.

STUDENT ACTIVITY

10.1 Design a wigroom order form suitable to be sent to a wigmaker. Discuss with your lecturer and colleagues what information you may require. You will need to include: client's name and reference number; enough space for the measurements to be recorded; the type and colour of hair together with a sample if possible; the style required; any abnormalities that may be present (cysts, etc.). You will also need the name of the person completing the form, the date the measurements were taken and the date the completed work is required; the price quoted; any additional details. Can you think of any more details required?

Your approach and attitude to the client is most important. This person may have been in an accident, or have lost his or her hair through illness and may be self-conscious. You should be discreet, tactful, sympathetic and professional throughout the consultation process and take the measurements in a quiet and confident manner.

The client should be seated comfortably in front of a mirror for the measuring session and you should explain what you are going to do and the reasons for accurate measuring. Drape a gown over the client.

Measurements required

- Circumference of head
- Forehead to nape
- Ear to ear (over crown)
- Ear to ear (top of head)
- Temple to temple around back of head
- Nape
- Ear arch to nape
- Temple to temple front hairline

Circumference of head

This is the total distance around the head. With a good dressmaking tape measure, start by measuring from just above the hairline at the centre front (about 1cm in from the hairline). Proceed around the head, at the same distance in from the hairline and take the measurement when the tape reaches its starting point.

Forehead to nape

Measure from centre front to centre back – going over the top of the head.

Ear to ear (over crown)

The ear peak, often referred to as the ear point or the ear front, is the point just in front of the ear. Measure from this point to the same point in front of the other ear. Pass the tape measure along the hairline as you do so.

Ear to ear (top of head)

Measure from the hairline above the topmost point of the ear, over the top of the head, to the same point above the other ear.

Temple to temple around the back of the head

Measure from the temple point around the back of the head, taking in the widest part of the head, around to the same position on the other temple.

TIP

Tape measures stretch with use. Use the same measure for drawing the pattern and measuring the pattern and mounting the wig.

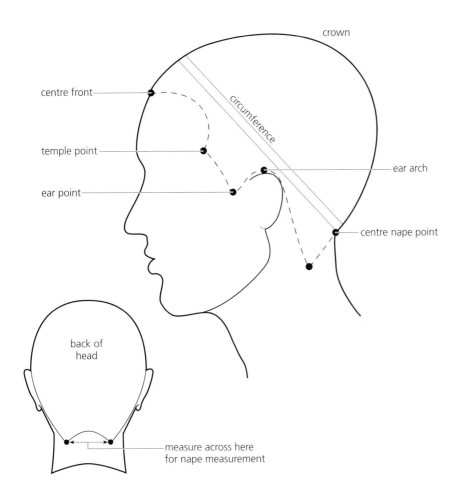

crown

centre front

temple point

ear point

circumference

ear arch

centre nape point

back of
head

measure across here
for nape measurement

Measurements for a wig

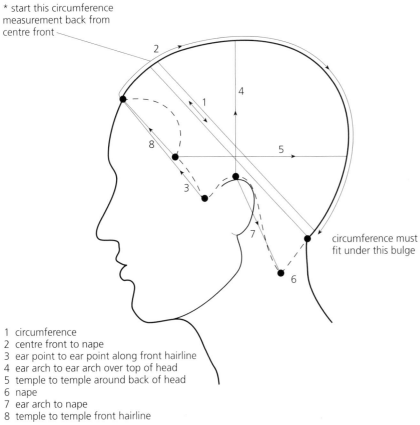

* start this circumference
measurement back from
centre front

circumference must
fit under this bulge

1 circumference
2 centre front to nape
3 ear point to ear point along front hairline
4 ear arch to ear arch over top of head
5 temple to temple around back of head
6 nape
7 ear arch to nape
8 temple to temple front hairline

Nape

Measure across the back of the neck.

Ear arch to nape

Measure from the ear arch to the corner nape point (see illustrations).

Temple to temple front hairline

**EQUIPMENT AND
PRODUCT LIST**

Equipment and materials for
making a wig pattern

Equipment

Pencil and ruler

Scissors

Completed model record card
with measurements

Materials

Tracing paper – length 70 cm,
width 30 cm

Adhesive tape

Making the template/pattern

1 Take the pre-cut tracing paper and fold down the middle lengthways. This fold represents the centre front.

2 Measure in from the centre front, half the circumference. This represents the centre back.

3 Measure in from the centre front, half the ear to ear across the front hairline measurement. This indicates the ear front.

4 Measure in from this point 5 cm.

5 Shape the front hairline.

6 Measure in from the centre back half the nape measurement.

7 Measure up at this point 2 cm.

8 Measure up at the ear front 3 cm.

9 Measure up at centre back 3 cm.

10 Join these together, to shape around the ear and to shape the nape.

11 Determine the depth of the mount. This depends on whether or not a parting is to be included. If there is a parting, then the depth will be the same as the length of the parting plus 2 cm. If there is no parting, the depth is normally 5 cm.

12 Draw in the back line.

13 Cut out the pattern.

14 Place the pattern onto the client's head to check the fit. Pleat, where necessary. Strengthen the edges with adhesive tape.

15 If the pattern is not to be used immediately, pad it out to retain its shape.

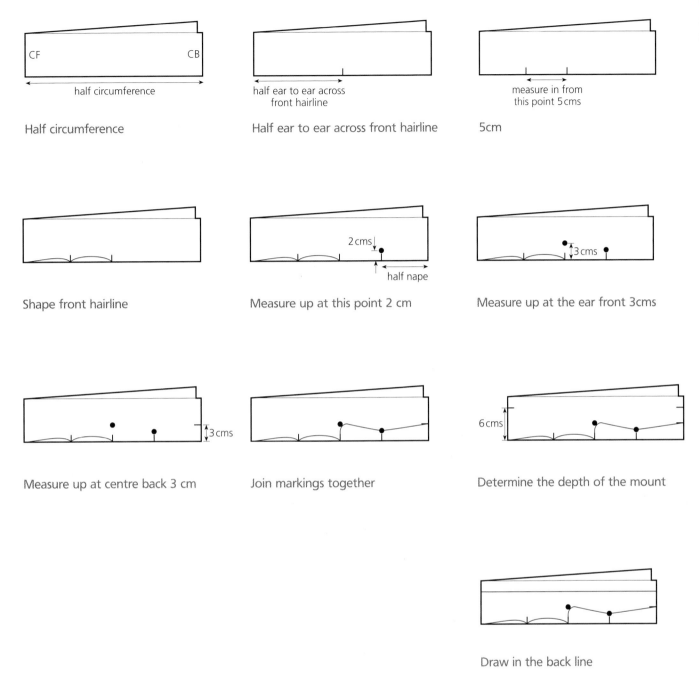

Half circumference

Half ear to ear across front hairline

5cm

Shape front hairline

Measure up at this point 2 cm

Measure up at the ear front 3cms

Measure up at centre back 3 cm

Join markings together

Determine the depth of the mount

Draw in the back line

Setting the wig or hairpiece

Setting the wig or hairpiece in the required style includes how to anchor the wig or hairpiece on a suitable block with tape and pins in order to work on it. The different sizes of block available for wigs and the importance of using the correct size block have to be known and understood. Products for setting and finishing the wig or hairpiece must be used appropriately.

Applying the wig or hairpiece

Wigs may be fitted with or without adhesive. You must be able to flatten the natural hair effectively, where necessary, and provide adequate anchorage for the wig or hairpiece. An even shape must result so that the wig or hairpiece appears as natural as possible. The wig/hairpiece must be fitted correctly and securely for the comfort and confidence of the wearer.

1 Seat the client comfortably and cover with a protective gown.
2 Make sure the area is adequately ventilated and all health and safety precautions have been taken into consideration to ensure compliance with the relevant legislation for the protection of the client as well as yourself.

HEALTH AND SAFETY

If the client has any history of allergies/intolerances or reactions to make-up solvents, a patch test is carried out 24 hours before application.

STUDENT ACTIVITY
10.2   Research sources of wigs and postiche for purchase and hire in your area.

POSTICHE WORK

Applying facial hair is important in period and historical make-up and can dramatically change the appearance of any character, particularly in theatrical ageing – see Chapter 11.

Types of hair used in postiche work

The most widely available hair is made from sheep's wool, but other animal hair, human hair and synthetic fibres are also available.

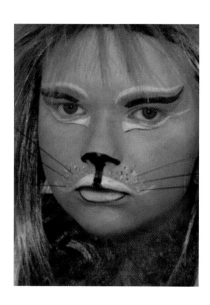

- *Wool crepe hair* – this is the cheapest type of hair, and comes braided over two strands of cord which are removed before using the hair. Wool crepe hair does not have long hairs, but consists of many shorter hairs, held together by overlapping. Wool crepe hair comes in many colours, with shades of blond, brown, black, grey, red and white. These look natural when mixed.
- *Real crepe hair* – braided together in the same way as wool crepe hair, but consists of human or animal hair. When the cords have been removed, the skeins (lengths) are usually 15 cm or 20 cm in length.
- *Angora goat hair* – also known as mohair, this is very soft and is usually used for fantasy work. It colours well, but is very expensive.
- *Yak hair* – naturally black, grey or off-white, and very coarse. It is particularly suitable for a stiff moustache or beard. It is sold by the ounce and is reasonably priced. It can be coloured.
- *Horsehair* – this hair is stiff and straight. It is often used for barristers' and judges' wigs. It is also useful for adding whiskers to an animal make-up – see Chapter 11, p182.

- *Human hair* – tends to be used solely for wigs and hairpieces.

- *Synthetic fibres* – wigs and hairpieces can be obtained as artificially created *plastic hairs*. Wigs and hairpieces made from synthetic fibres are more difficult to dress. However, it is tough and long lasting, so many rented wigs, for period work, are made of artificial hair. They are suitable for theatre productions but not used much in television or film work as they are less natural looking than real-hair work.

Applying facial hair directly to the skin

The main advantage of adding facial hair directly onto a model's face compared to a ready-made piece is that, if applied correctly, it can be almost impossible to tell it apart from natural facial hair. Always start by planning the work. Determine the shape and colours of the facial hair required. Be aware of the natural line of hair growth. Work to a picture or drawing and prepare a design sheet.

Preparing crepe hair

Crepe hair usually comes in plait form and can be bought in various lengths – the usual length to work with is 30 cm. Unwrap the crepe from the plait and remove string by cutting at the length you need. Once it is undone, the hair is curly or frizzy, so it must be straightened to make it workable. There are several ways of doing this:

- Damping the hair and leaving it stretched taught to dry will do this, but it takes time.

- Heavy weights can be placed over covered damp hair and left overnight.

- Heating – for speed, especially if you are applying facial hair with little or no notice, it is much more practical to use heat. First dampen the crepe hair, then, using either an iron or hair straighteners, gently pull the hair as you apply heat. This will straighten the hair quickly and effectively. Although crepe hair will withstand quite a high temperature, always check a small piece first.

TIP	

When working with crepe hair, keep your work area clean and tidy – crepe hair gets everywhere and you may get in a muddle.

Combing or hackling the hair

After straightening the hair it can be **hackled** or combed by hand. The traditional way of hackling hair is impractical if you are asked to do facial hair at short notice, so you will need to be able to use a comb as well. This whole process is time consuming but important, as it prevents clumps of hair in the final application. Eventually you will end up with a bundle of hair approximately 30 cm in length. Depending on the style of facial hair required, split the bundle into smaller sections. Each section is cut in half

---

EQUIPMENT AND PRODUCT LIST

Equipment and products used for laying on facial hair, using crepe hair, directly onto the skin

Equipment

Iron or hair straighteners or heavy weights

Wide toothed comb or hackle (p 159)

Scissors and tail comb

Small piece of damp towel

Products

Pre-bought crepe hair – in desired colour/s

Spirit gum and spirit gum remover

HEALTH AND SAFETY

When working with electrical appliances, always follow COSHH guidelines. Check equipment regularly and be careful with trailing leads.

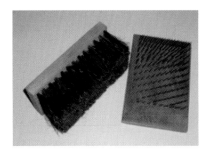

A hackle

diagonally, this angle is required to ensure the hair, once applied, looks like it is growing in a realistic direction – generally downwards for beards and backwards for head hair. If the hair is cut at a right angle, the effect will be to produce hair that sticks straight out from the face and looks fake.

A hackle is a piece of wood with a series of metal prongs set obliquely. These spikes are very sharp and the hackle should be clamped to a bench to comply with health and safety regulations. The function of the hackle is to free and disentangle the hair.

To hackle:

- Draw the hair through the teeth of the hackle a little at a time, in workable lengths, until it is knot free and smooth.
- When one side of the hair is free from tangles, turn it around and hackle the other side.
- Once hackled, hair can be stored on the hackle until ready to mix.
- After use, clean the hackle by drawing a comb across it, between the spikes, to remove any remaining hair, cover and put away in a safe place. It is essential to keep the spikes covered when not in use – and out of reach of children.

To comb:

Lay workable lengths of hair onto a towel on a flat surface and draw a large wide toothed comb through the hair until it is knot free and smooth. This can be laid on the towel in colours ready to mix.

Mixing the hair

Nobody has hair of just one colour, even 'black' hair has more than one colour. In order to look natural, the hair must be mixed. You can mix it on a hackle but it is easier and more practical to be able to mix by hand. Take small amounts of the colours you wish to mix between the thumb and forefinger of both hands and hold it firmly, but not too tightly, then pull the hair apart. Lay the bottom hair over the top hair and repeat, do this as many times as necessary until you have the required colour. To obtain a natural look, do not over blend or you may end up with a non-descript colour. Aim to create a sufficient blend that does not contain 'clumps' of colour.

Laying the hair

Once again it is important to keep your work area neat and tidy! Starting at the bottom of the area where the hair is to be applied, work upwards put a line of spirit gum (mastix) and wait for it to become tacky.

- *Beards* – lay the hair on in layers following the natural growth pattern (not all facial hair grows in the same direction). Hold the hair between the thumb and forefinger and roll it slightly, lay it against the spirit gum and press it into place with a piece of damp towel, this will prevent the hair and gum from sticking to you. Work methodically until you have covered the area required.
- *Moustache* – when working on a moustache the same rule applies, work in layers from the bottom upwards.

- *Sideburns* – to create sideburns you must first move your model's own hair out of the way, and comb the hair upwards with a fine tail comb or cutting comb, hooking it over the model's ear. Paint a thin layer of spirit gum in the desired shape of the sideburns. You can now lay on the hair in the same way as before, starting at the bottom and working upwards to meet the natural hair. If you are working on a man, he may already have sideburns to work up to, but on a female you will have to take the sideburns to the natural hair.

Dressing out

Once complete, trim and style the beard, moustache or sideburns as required. If changing a female to a male, you will have to add hair to the eyebrows too. This is done in the same way, working from the outside in and following the growth pattern. However be careful not to overdo it; only use a small amount of hair in this area and don't forget the bridge of the nose.

To remove:

Trim the hair close to the skin, and remove the hair using spirit gum remover (mastix remover) on a cotton wool pad, work from the top down until all the hair and spirit gum are removed. Finish by cleansing, toning and moisturising the skin.

Stubble

Stubble can quickly and easily transform a character. It is not always practical for an actor to grow his own stubble, and so it is often necessary to create some. Because filming is seldom done in the same order as the storyline, continuity often demands that the actor be both clean shaven and unshaven in the same day's work. If you are changing a female into a male, adding stubble will make the look very believable.

1 Pre-darken the beard area using a stipple sponge with grey/blue greasepaint, and powder well (optional).

2 Prepare the hair as before and cut it into even pieces approximately 2–3 mm long.

3 Using soft wax spread evenly over the face, and working on small areas at a time, follow the natural beard line. When applying stubble you must work from the top down so that you do not flatten the hair you have already applied.

4 Lay a small piece of pre-cut lace over the wax (make sure the lace is taught and pressed into the wax). Next, take your soft brush and, keeping it at a right angle to the dish, dip it into the hair and then lightly push the hair into the lace in the opposite direction to the natural hair growth (if the hair grows down then apply the hair in an upward direction).

5 Once you are happy that you have applied sufficient hair, slowly peel away the lace in the direction of growth (in this case down). Work in sections until you have completed the stubble area and make sure you take it down onto the neck as far as the Adams apple. Be careful not to touch any stubble you have already applied, as it will flatten it to the skin

EQUIPMENT AND PRODUCT LIST

Equipment and products used for making stubble

Equipment

Fine hair lace

Soft brush (preferably dome shaped)

Stipple sponge (optional)

Small dish

Scissors

Products

Short cut-up real hair (3 mm long)

Wax (stubble paste)

Grey/blue greasepaint (optional)

making it look unnatural. The hair should look like it is growing out from the skin.

6 If any small areas are missed, it may be necessary to apply more wax, lace and hair and go over the areas again.

To remove:

Remove hair by applying cleanser to the area and scraping the stubble off with either a spatula or a tissue. Finish by cleansing, toning and moisturising in the usual way.

Sex reversal – female to male

Start by pre-darkening the beard area with a grey/blue greasepaint, and a stipple sponge, and powder well. Apply stubble to required area, following the instructions above. When changing a female into a male, you may have to use make-up to shade and give a more 'manly' appearance, brown greasepaint was used to shade under the eyes and around the temples. To give a dishevelled look, Mehron 'Sweat and Tears' was applied over the nose and on the forehead to make her appear sweaty.

EQUIPMENT AND PRODUCT LIST

Equipment and products for female to male character change

Equipment

Stipple sponge

Wig lace (fine)

Soft brush (preferably dome shaped)

Small dish

Scissors

Products

Prepared crepe hair, 2–3 mm lengths cut and ready for use

Mehron 'Sweat and Tears' (optional)

Wax (stubble paste)

Grey/blue greasepaint (optional)

Spirit gum and remover

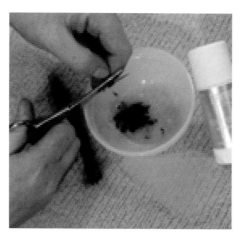
Hair being cut ready for applying

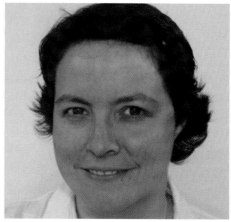
Gender change woman to man before

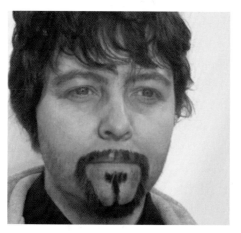
Gender change woman to man stage 1

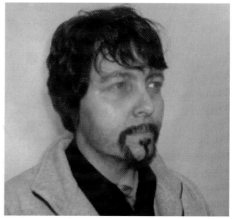
Gender change woman to man final

APPLYING FALSE EYELASHES – STRIP AND INDIVIDUAL

False eyelashes are an absolute must for all make-up artists' kit bags. They are invaluable when doing a 1960s or 1970s make-up and are often used in catwalk, pop video and editorial shots. False eyelashes can be made from threads of nylon fibre or real hair and come in all different shapes, sizes and colours. The lashes made from nylon fibre hold a permanent curl for a longer time than natural hair and are more cost effective than real hair lashes, which tend to be very expensive. False lashes are attached close to the model's natural lash roots, with adhesive on the eye lid, imitating the natural eyelashes and making the lashes appear longer and thicker, thereby drawing attention to the eye. There are two main types:

- Semi-permanent individual lashes – designed to be worn for approximately 4–6 weeks.

- Strip lashes – designed to be worn for a short period, either a day or an evening.

Using false lashes can:

- make natural lashes look longer and thicker
- add definition to the eye area
- enhance photographic make-up
- enhance an evening or fantasy make-up
- complete a corrective make-up – adding shape and depth
- provide an alternative eyelash-enhancing effect for a model who is allergic to mascara (providing they are not allergic to the adhesive used in applying them!).

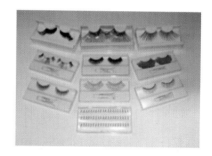

A selection of false eyelashes

Factors to consider when choosing lashes:

- The model's natural lashes. Does the model have short or long lashes? Sparse or thick? Curly or straight? Choose lashes that complement the natural lash, the model's hair and skin tone.

- The model's age: artificial lashes create a very bold, dramatic effect, which can make an older model look harsh. False lashes should enhance the model's appearance.

- The occasion for wearing false eyelashes: this can determine whether individual or strip lashes are more appropriate, for example individual for corrective, long-term use, or strip lashes for an evening out, a photo shoot or for a fantasy make-up.

- Maintenance of the lashes – strip lashes require little maintenance as no special product is needed for removal and they can be reused, making them a cost effective product. Individual lashes, however, need more maintenance. A solvent product is required to remove lashes and as natural lashes fall out, replacement false lashes need to be applied.

- Time – strip lashes are relatively easy to apply and may add a further 10 minutes to a make-up application time. Individual lashes on the other hand may add a further 30 minutes to make-up application time, depending on how many are applied.

Step-by-step instructions for applying semi-permanent lashes

Check that a patch test has been carried out and that there were no reactions to the adhesive being used.

Top lashes

1 After completing a full consultation with the model and deciding what length and colour lashes you will be using, prepare your trolley with everything you will need.

2 Prepare the model for treatment by wrapping hair in a turban or towel, removing jewellery and contact lenses if necessary and sitting model in a semi-reclined position with clothing covered.

3 Work from behind the model. Apply individual lashes with sterile tweezers. Hold the lash near the tip for extra support and for easier application. Apply adhesive, enough, but not too much to the underside of the lash. Using a stroking movement, place the underside of the false lash on top of the natural lash. As you line up the false lash for placement, slide the adhesive down the side of one of the natural lashes – 'guide' the false lash towards the base of the natural lash so that the false lash is resting along the length of the natural lash.

4 If you are applying lashes to the whole of the upper lid, start at the inner corner and work towards the outer corner, applying the shorter lashes to the inner corners and the longer lashes to the outer corners, to create a realistic effect. If you are applying lashes just to the outside corners, start at the outside and work inwards. To get both eyes exact, apply the false lashes one at a time, to each eye alternately. This also avoids working on one eye for too long a period – you don't want the model's eyes to start watering.

Bottom lashes

1 Work facing the model, with the model looking upwards, her eyes slightly open. Follow the same general procedure for applying lashes to the top lids, however, the lashes curve downwards and the adhesive is applied to the upper surface of the lash.

2 Use shorter lashes for application to the bottom lids for a natural look.

Step-by-step instructions for applying strip lashes

Check that a patch test has been carried out and that there were no reactions to the adhesive being used.

Top lashes

1 After completing a full consultation with the model and deciding what length and colour lashes you will be using, prepare your trolley with everything you will need.

2 Seat the model in a semi-reclined position and work from above.

3 Selecting the appropriate lash (strips are designed to fit either the right or the left eye), apply a fine film of adhesive to the base of the false lashes – making sure there is enough adhesive on the ends, as they tend to flick up without enough adhesive!

4 Using tweezers to hold the eyelash, place it gently onto the skin of the eye lid as close as possible to the model's lashes.

5 With firm but careful pressure, and using the tweezers and an orange stick, gently press the false lash into place. Hold the lash in place in the centre with tweezers, and press the lash with an orange stick along the natural lash line.

6 The model's eyes are closed throughout the application process. After a few seconds the model can open her eyes, and you can check that the placement is correct.

7 If it is not correct, remove immediately, before the adhesive has had time to adhere securely and try again.

8 When the lash is in place, continue with make-up application, applying eyeliner to further secure and hide the false lash roots and to give a professional finish to the make-up.

Bottom lashes

It is usually unnecessary to apply false strip lashes to the bottom lashes. However, in a stage situation, or for a cat walk show, fashion shoot or a 1960s or 1970s make-up, it may be necessary. Strip lashes for the bottom lids are finer than those for the top lid, and have an extremely fine base. Apply in the same way as for the top lashes.

> **HEALTH AND SAFETY**
>
> Lashes may need to be trimmed – especially for the inner corner of the eye. If inner lashes are too long, they may irritate the model's eye.

Make-up application

For individual semi-permanent lashes, the lashes are applied first and light eye make-up applied after. Do not use mascara, as this will reduce the adhesion to the natural lash. Mascara also clogs the lashes together, and is difficult to remove without affecting the eyelash adhesive.

For strip lashes, there is no hard and fast rule. Either the make-up can be completed and the lashes applied at the end, or the application of the strip lashes can be during the eye make-up procedure. With strip lashes, eyelash curlers can be used, and mascara can also be used to mix the natural lashes in with the false ones. Liquid eyeliner can be applied to hide any adhesive that may have escaped, which would give an unprofessional finish. Black adhesive is now available and is recommended for photoshoots.

Removal of semi-permanent individual lashes

1 Position your model on the couch and wash your hands.

2 Remove any make-up from the area with an oil-free eye make-up remover.

3 Protect the surrounding eye tissue by placing a pre-shaped eye shield underneath the lower lashes of each eye – to protect the area from the solvent. Position the eye shields as close to the base of the lower lashes as you can.

4 Have the model close her eyes and ask her not to open them again until you tell her to do so.

5 With a new cotton bud (one with a pointed end) or an orange stick with a little cotton wool around it, moisten with the eyelash adhesive solvent.

6 Treating one eye at a time, gently stroke down the false eyelash with the adhesive solvent until the adhesive dissolves and the false eyelash begins to loosen.

7 Supporting the upper lid with one hand, with the other hand gently remove the false eyelash with a sterile pair of tweezers. There should be no resistance. If there is, then apply solvent again. Never pull at the lashes as this will cause discomfort to the model.

8 As the artificial lashes are removed, collect them on a clean tissue.

9 When all the lashes are removed, soothe the area with dampened cotton pads to ensure that all the adhesive is removed. Repeat on the other eye.

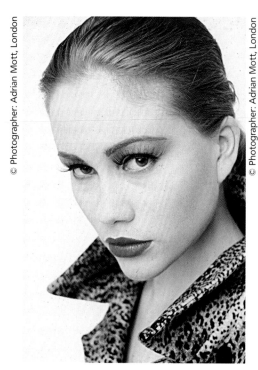

© Photographer: Adrian Mott, London

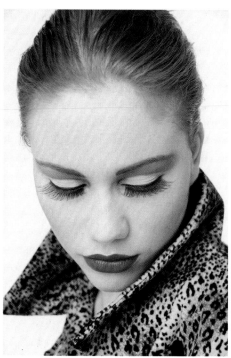

© Photographer: Adrian Mott, London

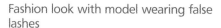

Fashion look with model wearing false lashes

Same fashion look photographed from a different angle – note the detail the camera picks up

Removal of strip lashes

1 Strip lashes need to be removed every night, and therefore the model will need instructions on how to do this. With clean hands, lift the strip from the outer corner of the eye. Supporting the eye with the other hand, gently peel the strip away from the natural lash, from the outer edge towards the centre of the eye lid.

2 Peel the adhesive from the backing strip using a clean pair of tweezers, trying to keep the lash in its original shape, and clean according to manufacturer's instructions.

3 Re-curl if necessary with eyelash curlers and store them in their original box.

Assessment of knowledge and understanding

Knowledge review

1 List the six pieces of equipment used when making a paper pattern.

2 Why is the record card needed during pattern making?

3 Give four measurements used when making a pattern for a wig.

4 What length should the paper be for the pattern?

5 What measurement is used for the front hairline?

6 What determines the depth of the mount?

7 How do you ensure you have a perfect fit?

8 What is the main reason for a workroom order form when ordering wigs?

9 Why is a photograph helpful to the wigmaker?

10 What is meant by abnormalities – give an example.

chapter 11

Theatrical and media make-up

Working in the theatre and media as a make-up artist requires both additional and different skills to those learned in Level 2. Level 3 work builds upon and often exaggerates the basic make-up techniques learned in Level 2, and introduces you to new techniques and products. The work includes special effects, where you will learn to work with wax and numerous varieties of stage blood. Ageing and character change make-up, as well as using ready made prosthetics, are all included in this chapter, and there is an introduction to making your own prosthetics, giving you a fantastic opportunity to use your imagination and let loose your creative talents in creating your own characters. The more experience and skills you have in these areas, the more employment opportunities will be open to you. It is best to gain this experience in the first instance by achieving formal qualifications. Building a college portfolio is an important start to your career and a great learning experience. Assisting in small theatres and amateur productions will also be invaluable, learning as much as possible in all areas.

Learning objectives

In this chapter you will learn about:

- special effects make-up:
  - working with wax
  - blocking out eyebrows
  - bruising, bullet wounds, scars, superficial cuts and grazes, scabs, deep cuts, and burns

- ageing:
  - male and female ageing with make-up
  - latex ageing
  - red stippled nose

- changing the appearance of a person:
  - gender reversal – male to female
  - gender reversal – female to male

- looks from hit musicals:
  - Bombay Dream
  - Madam Butterfly
  - Chicago
  - Cats

Learning objectives (cont.)

- historical figures:
  - Robin Hood and Maid Marion
  - Henry VIII
- fun figures
  - Betty Boop
- special effects for eyes using contact lenses
- bald caps
- prosthetics:
  - custom made prosthetics
  - how to apply ready-made prosthetics
  - werewolf make-up
  - Halloween characters
  - introduction to making your own prosthetics
- special effects for eyes
- clear instructions – pantomime vs. fashion

STUDENT ACTIVITY

11.1   Start making a collection of faces and characters to assist you in your theatrical make-up work. Collect old photographs and magazine cuttings of people of all ages and nationalities. Keep the pictures in a well organised scrapbook or photograph album with see-through sheets for easy reference. Examples include: characters from history and fiction; clowns; animal faces; faces and nationalities; unusual noses and eyes; aged males and females; happy and sad faces; bald and balding heads and beards and moustaches.

SPECIAL EFFECTS MAKE-UP

Ask anyone to describe 'special effects' and their definition may include sound effects, scenery, backdrops, props, lighting, clever computer graphics and make-up. This chapter, however, covers only the kind of special effects that can be achieved with make-up and the application of artificial parts (prosthetics). Special effects make-up includes casualty simulation make-up, which includes cuts and bruises, burns and bullet wounds. Other special effects include ageing, bald cap work, character change and the creation of all types of monsters and unusual characters with the use of prosthetics and postiche. Special effects help to make films, plays and TV dramas, especially hospital dramas, more visually spectacular.

Working with wax

Creating special effects with derma wax is very easy and it is the product most used in wound make-up. In a very short time you can create effects which, even at close range, look both realistic and gory. Derma wax, which is a kind of 'skin wax' is used to simulate disfigurements of the skin. Originally used by morticians – for concealing injuries on corpses to make the deceased look presentable at funerals – this wax comes in a range of different makes, each with their own unique colour and texture.

Grimas Derma Wax

A hard wax which requires a lot of pre-softening, for instance by mixing it with a rich moisturiser. It tends to be uneven in texture if not kneaded well enough before use. The wax is colourless and blends well with the natural colour of the skin.

Snazaroo wax

A medium-soft wax which tends to be of an uneven texture if not kneaded enough. The wax is of a strange yellowish colour and is easy to work with, although it is almost too soft at times.

Make-Up International Wax

Used for areas that have lots of movement. This wax is softer and doesn't 'lift' with movement.

Mehron Synwax

A hard wax which can withstand more pressure when you are colouring it.

Eyebrow wax

A hard wax that requires a lot of pre-softening. It tends to be uneven in texture if not kneaded well enough. This wax isn't dyed and blends well into the colour of the skin.

Blocking out eyebrows

You will often need to block out eyebrows in order to achieve specific looks. You can block out eyebrows to:

- Conceal their colour.
- To flatten the hairs against the skin so that they stay down for the duration of a performance.
- To remove, or to change their shape and/or size. Specific looks include clown or fantasy make-up and twentieth-century looks – 1920s (to straighten), 1930s and 1940s (to dramatically curve).

1 Cleanse the brows so they are free from any make-up and brush upwards so the hair is lying as flat to the skin as possible in one layer.
2 Using a modelling tool, scrape a small amount of wax from the container.
3 Hold the skin above the brows taught and, with the modelling tool, apply a thin layer of wax to the brows, in an upward direction, to ensure a flat smooth finish. Cover all the hairs including any between the brows if necessary.
4 Apply fixative.
5 Cover with desired foundation before creating new eyebrows for character change or specific era make-up.

EQUIPMENT AND PRODUCT LIST

Equipment and products to wax out eyebrows

Equipment

Eyebrow brush

Modelling tool

Products

Cleanser and toner

Grimas Eye Brow Plastic

Grimas Fixative 'A' sealer

Non-irritating soap

If you have no wax or plastic, then soap is a good standby. Cut some un-perfumed, non-irritating soap, into small pieces and place in a container with some water to soften. After cleansing the brows so they are free from grease, brush the softened soap on the brows covering well. Comb the brows flat, and slide a (clean) finger over them to smooth down. Dry the soap with a hair dryer, and repeat this process as many times as it takes to reach a smooth surface that covers the brows with a smooth screen of dried soap. When the soap is very dry, apply a film of sealer and spread beyond the soaped area. Cover with greasepaint or cream stick, blending carefully into skin edges to match foundation colour. Press powder into the make-up, removing excess carefully with a powder brush.

Other blocking out projects

You can also block out sideburns, temple hair and front hairlines. The larger the area, the more layers you may need, but always work only one layer at a time allowing the application to dry thoroughly between layers. The soap method is probably the best for the larger areas – blocking out hair from the hairline to the crown for example. Small areas such as eyebrows merely need sealing, whereas larger areas may need to have some very fine nylon stocking cut to shape and stuck down with spirit gum around the edges, before sealing. The stocking is then covered with soap, dried, covered with greasepaint and then powdered before applying foundation with a stipple sponge.

TIP

For easier application, the wax or plastic can be warmed on the back of the hand or between the index finger and thumb. Only do this if your hands are extremely clean!

HEALTH AND SAFETY

Always protect the model's eyes when using a hair dryer.

TIP

Eyebrow stencils, in all shapes and sizes, can be obtained on clear plastic sheets and are invaluable when remodelling eyebrows.

STUDENT ACTIVITY

11.2 **Block out practice.** Blocking out eyebrows, sideburns and hairlines well takes practice. Using different types of wax, practise as much as you can on as many different people as you can find.

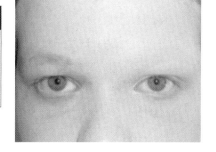

Blocking out eyebrows, before and after

HEALTH AND SAFETY

Caution with COSHH products, always carry out a patch test on models for sensitivity.

MAKE-UP ARTIST PROFILE: DORINDA SWEALES

How and when did you start in the business?

I started out training in beauty therapy in 1991, and achieved formal qualifications with VTCT in Theatrical and Media Make-up at Farnborough College of Technology. I specialised in make-up, as this was my love, and started with makeovers and bridal make-up, which led to work in theatre, television and photographic work.

Was there a turning point in your career?

There was no real turning point but having two children with special needs determined what kind of work I did. When I was asked to teach at Farnborough, it seemed the natural way to combine make-up with the time I needed to give my children. It also enables me to be picky about the freelance work I do as I have a regular source of income from teaching. Teaching is very satisfying and seeing a student's portfolio at the end of the year is fantastic, knowing that you have been an instrumental part of what they have achieved and seeing them complete the first steps on the road to where they want to be.

What do you consider to be important qualities for a make-up artist?

Firstly a passion for make-up is a must then in equal measures: good interpersonal skills, good organisational skills, patience, determination to succeed and pride in your appearance and your work. Oh, and the ability to work long hours and keep smiling!

What is your most memorable/exciting/best paid job?

Every new job is exciting but the most memorable are the *firsts*. The first bridal make-up; the first make-up in print; the first jobs in large theatres like the Royal Albert Hall and The Palladium (I love the atmosphere and the buzz of theatre and the fact that you are never quite sure how things will go); the first time working in a TV studio and the first time I taught, standing in for my old tutor. I'm a busy person and like to be on the go all the time so jobs where I have lots to do suit me best and I love working under pressure.

Have you had any disasters?

No, touch wood! But there have been occasions when I wished I'd had a product or piece of equipment with me that I'd thought I wouldn't need and had to improvise. This has taught me to be prepared and take things along that I may not need but may have cause to use unexpectedly or that someone else may need. I always have a bag of seemingly useless bits with me that come in handy for something!

What advice would you give to young people entering the industry?

Never give up, be determined and don't be put off by offhand comments made by others around you. Have faith in yourself and take time to tell yourself you are good at what you do. Some may tell you that your dreams are unreachable but my outlook on life is that you can achieve *anything* if you are willing to work hard to achieve it. When you start out don't turn work down because you think it is not taking you in the right direction. Very often from work you might have turned down comes other work which you will love. Meeting lots of people and networking is very important. JUST GO FOR IT ALL!

In your experience, would you advise those training to become make-up artists to specialise in one area only, or to gain experience, through Continued Professional Development courses (CPD) in many different areas of make-up?

I think it is important to train in a wide variety of areas, as only when you have covered all areas are you able to make the decision about where you want to specialise. Personally I like change so it is important for me to be able to work in different areas of make-up but I can understand why people specialise in one area. CPD is vital no matter what area of make-up you are in, there is always room for improvement as there are always new products on the market and new methods of application. You need to keep up to date to be competitive and offer a good service. Never fall into the trap of thinking you know it all. Our colleagues are also a vital source of new knowledge because we all work differently and you may find that the way someone else does something is actually quicker, easier or more effective. Life is one big learning curve take it all on board and use what you need to improve your skills. Above all, you have to continue to enjoy what you do.

Bruising

General bruise

All bruises are different, which makes them relatively easy to create. Avoid over-blending as the more time you spend 'playing' with the bruise the less realistic it will look. There are some considerations you must take into account when applying the make-up for a bruise:

- remember when creating bruises that there are no hard and fast rules
- no two bruises look the same and everyone bruises differently
- the cause of the bruise, the skin type and the age of the model will be governing factors in the way it looks.

The six main colours used in bruising are:

- red
- blue
- purple
- yellow
- brown
- green

These colours can be bought in one compact and are referred to as the 'bruise wheel of colours'. Once you have decided where the bruise is going to be and what has caused it, you must look at the age of the model and their skin type, do some research and get photographs of wounds on a similar aged person.

New bruises

1 Using either a sponge or your fingertips, apply red grease to the area to be bruised. This will give the effect of soreness.

2 Add a darker red to build up the colour and also some purple. Blend the colours, but do not over-blend, you do not want the bruise to look too uniform or it will be unrealistic. Make the impact areas darker (remember that the cause of the blow will determine the shape, you can use your brush for this) by using blue; this will also give the bruise depth. If the bruise is to be on an elderly person, then you may wish to use a little black grease.

3 Once complete you should powder the bruise to set it.

4 Apply a little petroleum jelly to it to give that swollen, just thumped look (optional).

To remove:

Remove products with cleanser, then tone and moisturise.

Old bruises

1 Using either a sponge or your fingertips, apply yellow to the area, then build up the bruise by adding green and brown and blend until you are happy with the effect. Again the cause and age of the bruise will determine the colours used.

EQUIPMENT AND PRODUCT LIST

Equipment and products for general bruising

Equipment

Selection of brushes and sponges

Product

Mehron bruise wheel containing red, purple, blue, yellow, brown and green

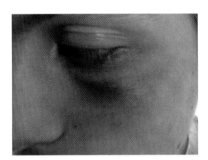

'Old' black eye bruise

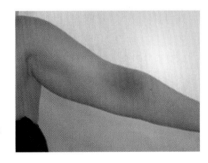

'Old' bruise on arm

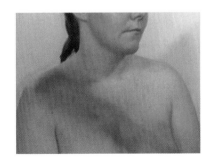

'Old' bruise – resulting from a seat belt

2 When you are happy with the look – powder to set it.

To remove:

Remove products with cleanser, then tone and moisturise.

Step by step bruising to the ankle

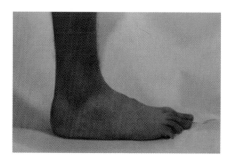
Bruising to the ankle before

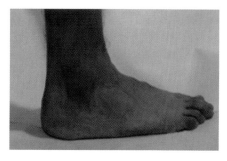
Bruising to the ankle sequence 1

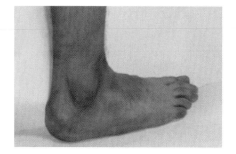
Bruising to the ankle sequence 2

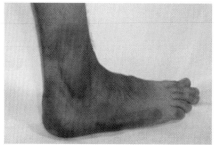
Bruising to the ankle sequence 3

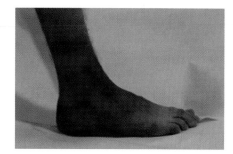
Bruising to the ankle final

Bullet wounds

EQUIPMENT AND PRODUCT LIST
Equipment and products for a bullet wound
Equipment
Selection of brushes and sponges
Products
Spirit gum
Synwax
Snazaroo cake blood
Grimas black grease
TTK congealed blood paste
Charcoal powder
Mehron Stage blood (dark)

Before you start, you will need to decide what kind of gun was used, what calibre it was and the distance it was fired from. Bullet wounds come in many shapes and sizes, some small and some large, and they can also be a variety of shapes. The angle the gun was fired from will also determine the shape of the wound. If you are asked to produce a bullet wound, find out the type of gun, research that particular type of gun and the wounds it is likely to produce, and use appropriate colouring to the wound as needed. The example shows a very quick and simple bullet wound, as would be made if hit by a .22 calibre gun.

1 Make sure that the area to be worked on is cleansed and toned but not moisturised, so that the adhesive will stick.

2 Apply a small amount of spirit gum to the area of the wound, whilst you are waiting for it to become tacky, take a small piece of Synwax and soften it between your fingers to make it workable, making sure that there are no lumps in it. Roll it into a ball and apply it to the adhesive (spirit gum).

3 Blend off the edges so that they are not visible.

4 Once you are happy with the wound, you can apply colour to it. Depending on the area of the body and the age of the wound you need to decide whether there will be any redness around it. If you wish to make it sore you should do so now using Snazaroo cake blood.

5 Using the black grease and the small brush, paint the bottom of the wound black, this will give it depth.

6 Next take the congealed blood paste and fill the wound.

7 Take a clean small brush and add a little charcoal powder to the edge of the wound. Once this is done you can add some blood. The amount of blood you use will be determined by the size of the wound and whether the subject is alive or dead. Large wounds on a live subject will have lots of blood, whereas a shot to the head killing instantly would not result in as much.

To remove:

Scrape off the excess wax, use spirit gum remover to clean away the spirit gum and cleanse, tone and moisturise in the usual way.

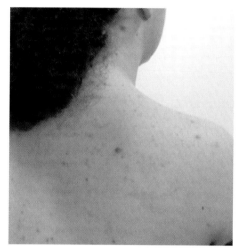
Bullet wound to shoulder before

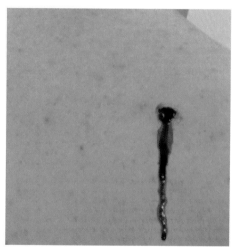
Bullet wound to shoulder after

Deep scar to the face

1 Apply a barrier cream and give it a few minutes to settle before you start.

2 Press the wax onto the area of the wound, making sure that the wax cylinder isn't too high. Massage the edges with a little rich moisturiser, to make the transition to the skin less obvious.

3 Draw a fine line with the red pencil (this would be for a recent scar, use white for an old scar) smudging it off at the ends. Paint on several thin coats of Rigid Collodion, waiting for each coat to dry before applying the next. You can use up to six coats to get a deep scar like the one in the example.

To remove:

Gently pick off the skin, then use spirit gum remover or acetone on any residue. Cleanse, tone and moisturise in the normal way.

EQUIPMENT AND PRODUCT LIST
Equipment and products for a deep scar
Equipment
Selection of brushes and sponges
Red pencil
Products
Cleanser and toner
Barrier cream and moisturiser
Synwax
Rigid Collodion

THEATRICAL AND MEDIA MAKE-UP

TIP ✔

Vaseline – when working with wax use a small amount of petroleum jelly (Vaseline) on your fingers and tools, this will prevent the wax from sticking and makes it easier to blend but be careful not to use too much. To prevent shine on your wax you should powder it gently using a colourless/transparent/translucent setting powder.

HEALTH AND SAFETY ✚

Rigid Collodion is a safe product to use, whereas flexible Collodion contains harmful ingredients and should be avoided.

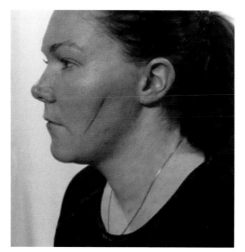

Face scar sequence 1

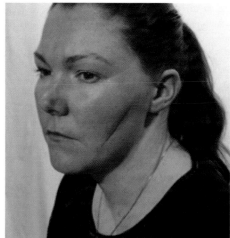

Face scar final

Cuts and grazes

Small cuts to the hand from barbed wire

1 Cleanse and tone the area to be worked on but do not moisturise, otherwise the adhesive will not stick.

2 Apply a small amount of spirit gum, depending on where the cuts are to be placed. Decide on the wax you are using and take a tiny amount to soften in your fingers then, using the modelling tool, spread the wax over the spirit gum making sure that the edges are well blended (remember that the wax is only there to make the cut and should not be visible).

3 Once you are happy with the wax, powder it using either a small brush or the edge of a make-up wedge.

4 Now you can make the cuts using the modelling tool. Carefully draw the line through the wax so that you do not lift it, then add some dark blood using your fine brush to paint it inside the cut. For the small hole you will have to decide on the angle at which the wire entered the skin, then, in the same way, apply the wound to the skin but keep the wax in a small round shape. Once it is blended and powdered, insert the tip of your modelling tool into it in the direction you have chosen, being careful not to damage it when you pull the tool out. Now you can insert the blood using your brush in the same way as before, this will give the impression that the blood is under the skin.

EQUIPMENT AND PRODUCT LIST

Equipment and products for barbed wire cuts

Equipment

Selection of sponges and brushes

Modelling tool

Fine brush

Products

Cleanser and toner

Spirit gum

Synwax

Setting powder

Mehron stage blood (dark)

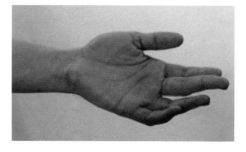

Small cuts by barbed wire before

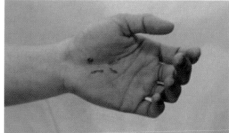

Small cuts by barbed wire after

To remove:

Scrape off the excess wax, use spirit gum remover to clean away the spirit gum, then cleanse, tone and moisturise in the usual way.

Bottle in face

1 Cleanse and tone the skin but do not moisturise, as this will prevent the spirit gum from adhering to the skin.

2 Ask your model to close their eyes and very carefully apply a small amount of spirit gum to the eye lid and onto the bridge of the nose. Take care not to get any in the eye, and whilst you wait for it to become tacky, take some wax in your fingers and roll it to make it smooth and workable.

3 Apply the wax to the closed eye lid – just following the natural shape of the eye. You need to have a layer around 2 mm thick to create the swollen look and it should be thicker at the centre, near and on the nose. Make sure that your edges are blended into the skin and not visible. Then cut into the thicker wax starting from the bridge of the nose and bringing it down the inner corner of the eye to give the effect of a flap of cut skin.

4 Apply wax to the side of the nose in the same way, blending it over the nose, down onto the cheek and up to meet the wax by the eye. As above, this is to give a swollen effect on the side of the nose. Make a cut in the wax at the bottom of the nose near the nostril to make it look as if it has been split.

5 Make sure that all your edges are well blended and not visible.

6 Using your wax in the same way, create cuts of differing sizes over the appropriate areas of the face that would have been cut by the bottle – again blending the edges out.

7 Once you are happy with the wax, you can start to apply colour. Start with the Snazaroo cake blood, building the colour up on the swollen areas, using less around the small cuts. You can add a small amount of the Grimas blue/black to the corner and under the eye, but be careful not to

EQUIPMENT AND PRODUCT LIST
Equipment and products for superficial cuts to the face
Equipment
Selection of sponges and brushes
Products
Cleanser and toner
Spirit gum
Snazaroo cake blood
Grimas blue/black grease
Setting powder
Vaseline
Mehron stage blood (dark)

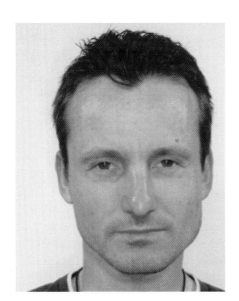

Superficial cuts to the face before

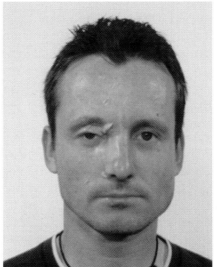

Stage 3, 4 and 5 – apply wax to eyelid, side of nose and onto cheek

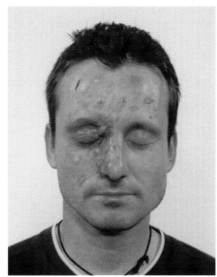

Stage 7 – apply colour to cuts and under eye

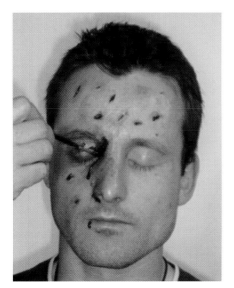

Apply colour to corner of eye

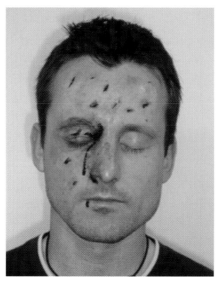

Set make-up. Apply vaseline to swollen areas

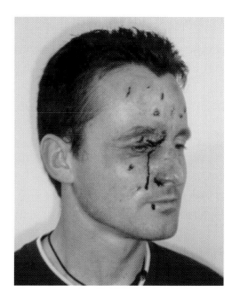

Superficial cuts to face – final

make it look bruised. Your aim is for impact marks rather than bruises, as it is a fairly new wound.

8 Once the colour is complete, set the make-up with powder then use Vaseline over the swollen areas to emphasise the effect. Also do this around cuts that are in prominent areas.

9 Finally, using your small brush, carefully apply a little blood to the small cuts and a bit more to the larger ones. Think about the position your subject would be in, as this will determine the direction that the blood will run. You may need to apply the blood in situ.

To remove:

Very carefully scrape away the excess wax before cleansing the area around and above the eye using adhesive-removing cream, as this will not drip into the eye. Ordinary spirit gum remover may be used on the lower areas of the face if required. Once spirit gum is removed you can cleanse, tone and moisturise in the normal way.

Graze to elbow

To create sore redness, use a damp make-up sponge and Snazaroo cake blood and Mehron coagulated blood using a black stipple sponge. Sweep it across the skin in the direction you want the graze to be, remembering that grazes tend to occur more on bony prominences. The effect of grit is made by mixing coffee granules with a small amount of congealed blood paste and applying it with a small brush. Grazes are best kept simple, the less time you spend on them the more realistic they look, so don't over do it.

To remove:

Cleanse, tone and moisturise in the normal way.

EQUIPMENT AND PRODUCT LIST

Equipment and products for a graze to the elbow

Equipment

Selection of sponges and brushes

Products

Snazaroo cake blood

Mehron coagulated blood

Coffee granules

TTK congealed blood paste

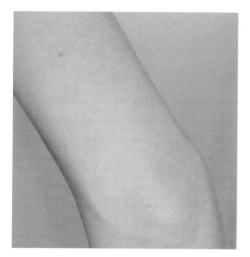

Graze on elbow before

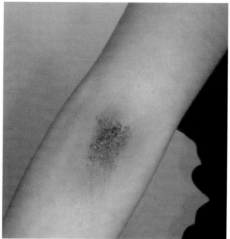

Graze on elbow after

Scab on chin

This technique can be used on any area; for smaller scabs, maybe around the mouth, you would need to make sure the bran flakes are crushed finely. Choose a wax that is soft so it will not lift with movement.

1 Cleanse and tone the area but do not moisturise, as this will prevent the adhesive from sticking.

2 Use a damp sponge and the Snazaroo cake blood to redden the area slightly.

3 Apply a thin layer of spirit gum and wait until it becomes tacky before taking your modelling tool to apply wax to the area. Spread it evenly, it doesn't need to be too thick, just thick enough to push the bran flakes into.

4 Crush the bran flakes to make them small, then push them into the wax, making sure that the whole of the wax area is covered with the flakes.

5 When they are stuck you can begin to colour them by using the small brush and the Grimas black grease. Use this sparingly to paint over the flakes, as you do not want it to look too black.

6 Take some congealed blood paste and the small brush and paint over the scab making sure that the whole area has a thin coat, it is important that the scab does not look wet.

7 The scab can be left like this or, as in the photograph, it can be picked and made to bleed. Do this by using the end of the brush or the end of a modelling tool to pick out a small piece of the scab.

8 Finally add a small amount of Mehron dark blood.

To remove:

Gently scrape the wax and bran flakes away then remove spirit gum with spirit gum remover. The area can now be cleansed, toned and moisturised in the normal way to remove any remaining make-up.

EQUIPMENT AND PRODUCT LIST

Equipment and products for a scab on the chin

Equipment

Selection of sponges and brushes

Products

Cleanser and toner

Snazaroo cake blood

Spirit gum

Synwax

Bran flakes – crushed

Grimas black grease

TTK congealed blood paste

Mehron dark blood (optional) for picked scab

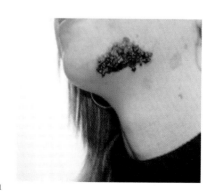

Scab on chin

Deep cut to thigh

The way the blood will run is dependent on the position the model is in. Remember to think of the way the wound has been caused. Most wounds will be deeper at one end than the other and may have flaps of skin overhanging at one end, which can be done with the wax. Remember to research every look. In this motor cycle accident, you may wish to apply bits of leaf or tree bark to the wound for authenticity.

1 Cleanse and tone the area to be worked on, but do not moisturise. This is to enable the spirit gum to adhere to the skin.

2 Apply spirit gum to the areas of the wound.

3 Whilst you are waiting for it to become tacky, take some Synwax and soften it in your hands. Make sure that it is soft enough to blend and has no small lumps in it. Roll it into a sausage shape before flattening it slightly, and placing it onto the spirit gum.

4 Using your modelling tool, blend it out to the sides so that you are making an open, almost rectangular shape. Raise the edges and make them jagged – the wound needs to be open but the jagged edges that are raised need to be turned in slightly to be realistic. Taper one end a little; this will become the end of the wound.

5 Once you are happy with the wax, apply the Snazaroo cake blood around the edges of the wound, using the edge of a sponge. Don't take the redness too far from the wound as it is a new wound.

6 Take a little black grease on a small brush and apply it to the bottom of the wound to add depth to it.

7 Using the small brush again, paint some congealed blood paste on the raised edges of the wound. Take the small dish and place some congealed blood paste into it and add a small amount of cotton wool. Mix together until the cotton wool is completely soaked. This can now be carefully spread inside the wound, filling it, giving the effect of bloody flesh.

8 Before adding the runny blood, you should use your green and brown grease or cake make-up and dirty down the area around the wound (if you are using grease remember to set it with powder). You are now ready to add your blood.

To remove:

Scrape off the excess wax and the cotton wool mix, remove the spirit gum with spirit gum remover, then cleanse, tone and moisturise in the normal way.

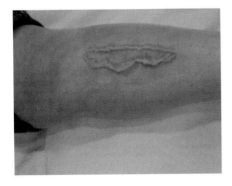

Stages 1, 2, 3 and 4 – apply wax and blend at sides

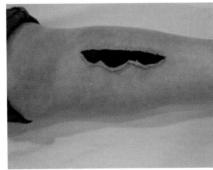

Stage 5 – apply cake blood

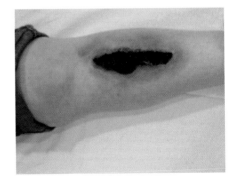

Stage 6 – apply black grease

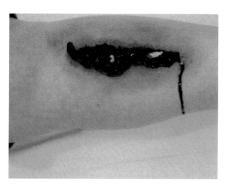
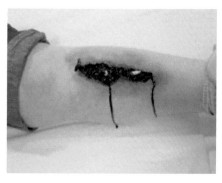

Stage 7 and 8 – apply congealed blood paste to raised edges of wound

Stage 8 – add runny blood. Deep cut to leg – final

Burns

Third degree burn to the sole of the foot using latex

1 Using the cake blood and a slightly dampened sponge, cover the entire foot area taking it up around the edges of the foot and a little way on to the ankle.

2 Pour a little latex into the dish and replace the lid on the bottle. Dip the sponge into the latex and cover the base of the foot.

3 Place the torn tissue over the foot, scrunching it slightly. Cover this completely with another layer of latex – making sure that all the tissue is soaked. You can do this a couple of times in the areas that would be most heavily burnt in order to build up the burn.

4 Once the latex is dry, use a sponge to give it a coat of cake blood.

5 Over this, apply the black grease, covering most of the area, but leaving a little of the red showing through. Take it around the edge of the foot and up the ankle a little way.

6 Now take the pointed end of your modelling tool and tear the latex in prominent places to expose the tissue underneath, open the tears up slightly making some larger than others, and cover this with the cake blood.

7 Fill the larger tears with a mix of cotton wool and congealed blood paste to look like deep burnt flesh. (Do not make the mix wet as the burn would be quite dry – you are aiming for a char-grilled effect).

8 Fill the smaller tears with congealed blood paste and the tissue will act as the flesh.

9 Take the beige from your burn wheel and, with a sponge and/or small brush, add some to the prominent areas and around the edges of the torn latex. Once you are happy with the look of the burn, use the Mehron Charred Ash powder to the burn and up around the edges of the foot and the ankle.

10 Finally, give the burn a fine mist of the glycerine and water mix.

To remove:

Wet the edges of the latex with cotton wool and warm water, gently working over the entire latexed area to lift it. If working on an area that is hairy, care must be taken to soak well. Once the latex has been removed, you can cleanse, tone and moisturise in the normal way.

EQUIPMENT AND PRODUCT LIST

Equipment and products for a burn to the sole of the foot

Equipment

Selection of sponges and brushes

Cotton wool

Modelling tool

Tissues

Products

Mehron burn wheel

Snazaroo cake blood

Liquid latex

Grimas black grease

TTK congealed blood paste

Mehron Charred Ash powder

Glycerine and water

TIP

Always replace the lid on the latex bottle, otherwise it will dry around the top of the bottle creating a solid plug.

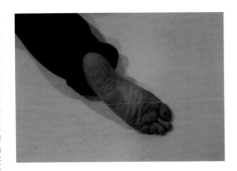

Foot without burn before

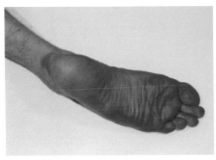

Stage 1 and 2 – apply cake blood and latex

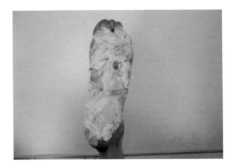

Stage 3 – apply torn tissue over foot, before applying more latex

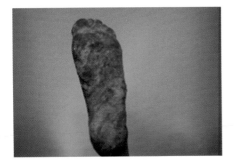

Stage 4 – apply a coat of cake blood

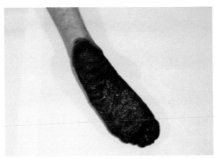

Stage 5, 6, 7 and 8 – tear latex in prominent places. Fill with congealed blood and cotton wool. Apply charred Ash powder

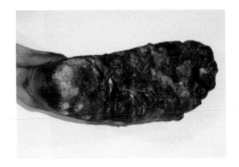

Apply mist of glycerine and water mix – final look

First and second degree sunburn

EQUIPMENT AND PRODUCT LIST
Equipment and products for first and second degree sunburn
Equipment
Selection of sponges and brushes
Surgical tape and scissors
Make-up sponge wedge
Modelling tool
Products
Mehron cake make-up in Starblend Red
Dark red grease or cake make-up
Tuplast (scar plastic) or gelatine or Mehron 3D Gel
Setting powder (optional)
Vaseline

To create strap marks, use tape to cover the skin that would have been under the strap.

1 Cut a wide piece of tape vertically down the middle. Stick one piece of the cut tape onto the skin with the cut edge on the neck side.
2 Then place the other piece of cut tape halfway over the first piece. This time with the cut edge on the arm side.
3 You are now left with two perfectly straight edges.

Once the tape is secure, you can apply the red to the area using your sponge, use the colour sparingly at first, as it is easy to apply more, but not so easy to remove when you have applied too much. First degree burns are not severe so don't over-do the red. Prominent areas catch the sun more, so apply a little more colour to the top of the shoulder. Once you are happy with the colour you can remove the tape carefully to reveal the strap mark. If you have used grease you will have to set it with powder. Finally, you may want to apply a tiny amount of Vaseline to prominent areas.

A second degree burn is done in the same way as the first degree burn, but the redness is more severe. You do this by applying a little of the darker red over the original red. Use the Tuplast straight from the tube, squeezing out different sized amounts to create blisters, shaping them with the modelling tool before it is dry. (Remember that not all blisters are the same size and shape.) Apply a little more redness over the top of the blisters. As an alternative to Tuplast, you could use gelatine or Mehron 3D gel.

To remove:

Gently peel off the blisters then cleanse, tone and moisturise in the normal way.

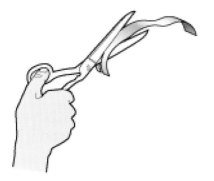

Stage 1 – scissors cutting tape vertically

tape overlapped

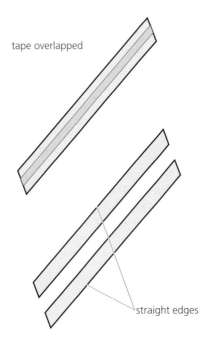

straight edges

2nd piece of tape

tape on shoulder with straight edges to outside

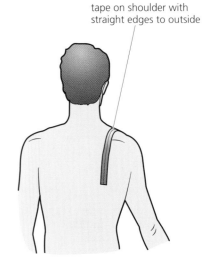

Two perfectly straight edges

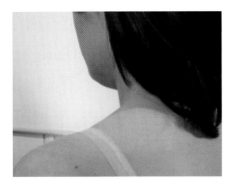

First and second degree sunburn – apply tape to required thickness

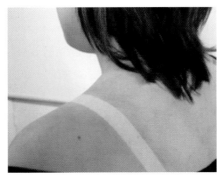

Stage 2 – apply red to whole area creating a first degree burn

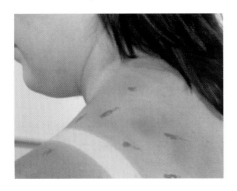

To create a second degree burn, apply a darker red over the original red and create blisters

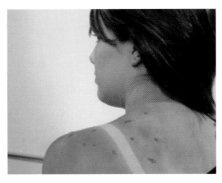

Stage 2 – apply more red over blisters

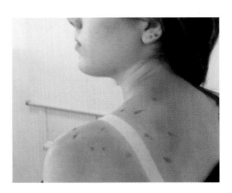

Second degree sunburn

EQUIPMENT AND PRODUCT LIST

Equipment and products for a chemical burn to the face

Equipment

Selection of sponges and brushes

Surgical tape

Modelling tool

Products

Mehron 3D gel

Mehron cake make-up in Starblend Red

Gelatine and water

TIP ✔

If your model, male or female, has facial hair, then wet the gel to soften it before trying to remove it.

Third degree chemical burn to the face using 3D gel

First think about the area you are working on and how the burn would have occurred. In this example, the burn is taken into the hair. Use tape over the hair for small areas, to make it look like the hair has been burnt away. For larger areas a bald cap would have to be applied, to which you can later add crepe hair on a hair-piece.

1 If working over the eyes, ears or part of the mouth, cover with surgical tape, to protect these sensitive areas.

2 By following the manufacturer's instructions, heat the 3D-gel to a working temperature, making sure it is not too hot. You will have to work quickly before the gel thickens. Squeeze the gel in a random pattern over the face, using your modelling tool to lift and criss-cross the gels whilst spreading, this will create holes and indents of varying sizes. You may have to heat the gel again, and add more. Do this until you are happy with the look.

3 Take the red cake make-up or grease and cover the whole area extending it beyond the area of the gel and onto the natural skin.

4 Add some cake blood or darker red grease in areas where you want to add depth, followed by the beige from the bruise wheel, which you should apply with a small brush in raised areas especially around the edges of the holes.

5 Take the congealed blood paste and a small brush and paint this into the holes and depressions.

6 Add some blood to the larger holes, but don't over do it.

7 Finally, if required, you should now add a spray of glycerine and water mix.

To remove:

Gently lift the gel away from the skin, being careful not to catch any fine facial hair. You can now cleanse, tone and moisturise in the normal way.

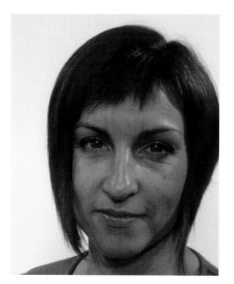

Chemical burn to face before

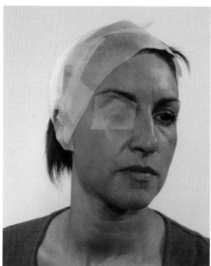

Stage 1 – protect hair and eyes with surgical tape

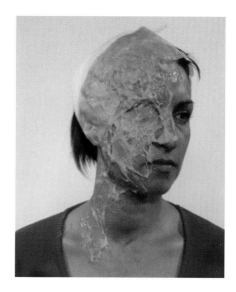

Stage 2 – apply gel, creating holes and indents of various sizes

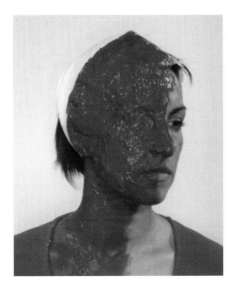

Stage 3 – cover white area with red cake make-up, overlapping onto natural skin

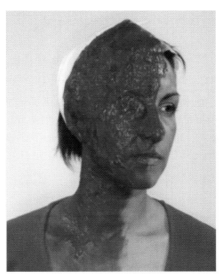

Stages 4, 5 and 6 – add darker red to add depth, beige to the raised areas and congealed blood to holes and depressions

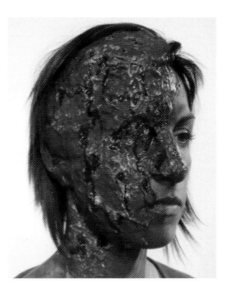

Stage 7 – spray with glycerine and water mix

AGEING

The two principal techniques of ageing are shading and highlighting. Shading should be used to make a feature less noticeable and highlighting to draw attention to features. There is no hard and fast rule about which you should apply first, the shading or the highlighting. Shading and highlighting follow the same techniques as corrective make-up, but instead of just correcting shadows and unwanted lines, these are deliberately exaggerated. The bone structure does not change in the ageing process, but the muscles around it become less elastic and fall to create wrinkles.

TIP

When creating a character, which requires ageing, remember that lines going down suggest age and lines going up suggest youth.

STUDENT ACTIVITY

11.3 Revise the muscles of facial expression in Chapter 2.

How strong the make-up needs to be will depend on the production. For a theatre production, the make-up can be quite obvious from the front of the theatre, as it needs to be seen at the back. For TV and film, make-up has to be blended very carefully so that it is not obviously make-up.

- Shading removes colour by taking back, causing the receding of shape. Shading should be carefully applied and the edge always blended with the base make-up so that there are no hard lines. Note that if shading is too strong, it can always be reduced by carefully stippling over with foundation colour.

- Highlighting adds colour by bringing forward and making features stand out. Therefore highlight the prominent features first.

Male and female ageing

The following examples of male and female ageing have been designed for stage work, to be seen at a great distance and under very strong lights.

It is usual to choose a foundation about two tones darker than natural complexion colour, in order for the highlighting and shading to be seen. However, if the model's skin colour is suitable for the character being portrayed, then select a foundation for the model's normal colour.

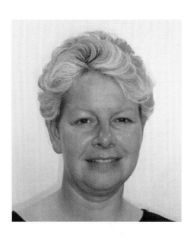

Female ageing before

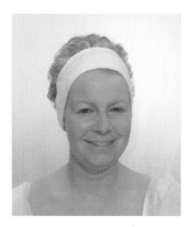

Stage 1 – preparing the model for make-up. Apply foundation two tones darker for highlighters and shaders to be seen

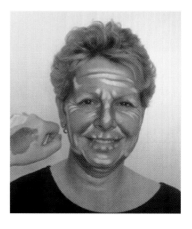

Stage 2 – mix appropriate highlight and shade colours, and apply to forehead, around eyes and mouth – depending on what facial expressions you want to achieve

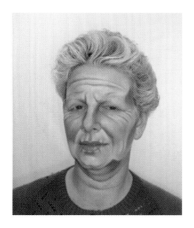

Stage 3 – continue with highlighting and shading until you have achieved the desired result

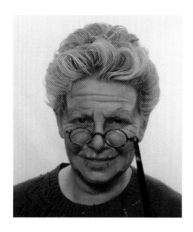

Female ageing final

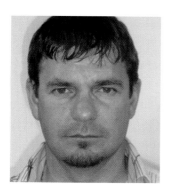

Male ageing before

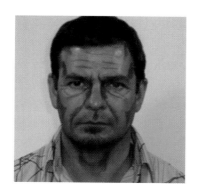

Stage 1 – preparing the model for make-up. Apply foundation two tones darker for highlighters and shaders to be seen

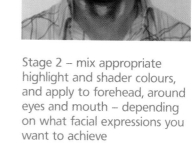

Stage 2 – mix appropriate highlight and shader colours, and apply to forehead, around eyes and mouth – depending on what facial expressions you want to achieve

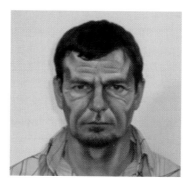

Stage 3 – continue with highlighting and shading until you have achieved the desired result

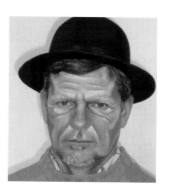

Male ageing final

Latex ageing

If ageing make-up alone is inadequate, liquid latex is sometimes used to age the face. When using latex, you will have to decide whether it is going to be sufficient to use it just around the eye area to make your subject middle-aged or whether you are going to age them vastly and apply it to the whole face. Take care when doing the whole face, as your model may look like they are wearing a mask. Only use a little product at a time, as it dries quickly and will become unworkable. If you need to colour the latex, it is done in the preparation stage before being applied to the skin. If you are working on a model with a dark skin tone, you can either add a dark powder or some pigment and always make sure the colour is well mixed.

When working with latex, the wrinkles will form in the *opposite* direction to the way you have stretched the skin. A horizontal stretch will result in vertical wrinkles and vertical stretching will result in horizontal wrinkles. Look at pictures of elderly faces to see how wrinkles form on the face. Decide where you want your wrinkles by drawing on paper first, and then use that as a pattern. If you are significantly ageing a model then you will want to age the hair and eyebrows, this can be done in the same way as you

TIP

Make sure your fingers are powdered before you start, so that you do not stick to the latex.

TIP

You will require help when applying liquid latex. One person will need to hold the skin taut, as another applies the product.

EQUIPMENT AND PRODUCT LIST

Equipment and products for latex ageing

Equipment

Selection of sponges and brushes

Hairdryer

Products

Barrier spray or mousse (oil free)

Setting powder

Liquid latex

Colour – optional

Brown mask cover

White grease paint

TIP ✔

When the latex has become transparent, it is dry.

TIP ✔

Remember to always replace bottle tops. This is particularly important with latex as the liquid becomes solid very quickly when exposed to the air.

---

would age hair and brows for stage ageing (see male and female examples above).

1 Protect the model's clothing by placing a protective cover around the shoulders.

2 Apply a barrier spray or mousse, making sure it is an oil-free brand, and then powder to remove all traces of grease.

3 Pour a little latex into the bowl, and colour if required.

4 Start at the top of the face, working in one section at a time. By stretching the forehead upward and the eyebrows downward you will create vertical lines across the forehead, apply the latex using a sponge using a stippling motion. (You will have to change sponges regularly as it will become clogged quickly.)

5 Once you have applied a layer of latex, dry it with the hairdryer, and then immediately powder it *before releasing the stretch*. You can apply up to three layers of latex on the forehead, drying and powdering between each, then work in sections down the face.

6 You can apply up to three layers all over the face and neck but make sure that you only apply one layer to the eye lids and underneath the eyes, making sure you powder before you release the stretch so that the latex does not stick to itself. Make sure that you take the latex right up to, but not into the hairline, and up to but not into the lashes.

7 When you have completed your application of latex, you may want to apply broken veins on the cheeks and nose using the stipple sponge and red mask cover – for more impact.

8 Apply age spots and/or moles using the brown mask cover with a small brush.

9 Ask the model to pucker their lips and dab on the white or very pale grease to make the lips look old and wrinkled.

TIP ✔

If you have aged a model's face, remember you may have to age the hands too.

HEALTH AND SAFETY ✚

Do not overload the sponge or the latex will drip into the model's eyes. Discard the sponges after use.

To remove:

To remove latex from the face you will need a towel to cover your model, a bowl of warm water and cotton wool. Soak the cotton wool in the water and wipe it against the edges of the latex to lift it. Work over the face gently, lifting the latex with the water. Never pull the latex from the skin and be careful of fine facial hairs because if the latex is not soaked it will pull on them and may cause pain. Once the latex is removed then you can cleanse, tone and moisturise in the normal way.

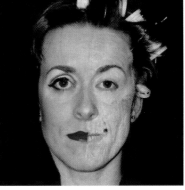

Latex ageing

Red stippled nose

Ageing need not just be the insertion of lines. This red stippled nose is a good example of an alternative method of ageing a gentleman. Stippling is one term used for applying face and body paint, or make-up onto the skin's surface. It is the continuous dabbing of the paint from the sponge to the face/body, which leaves the effect of a mottled/speckled finish to the skin.

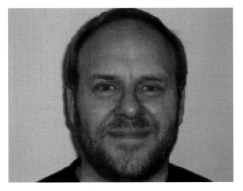

Model before stippling

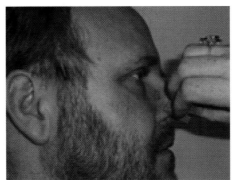

Stage 1 – using stippling sponge apply red make-up to nose area

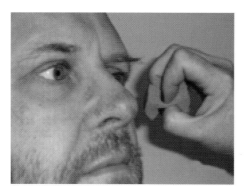

Stage 2 – continue stippling until you reach desired effect.

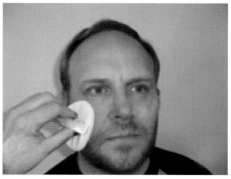

Stage 3 – applying foundation and setting with powder to cheeks will emphasise stippled nose more. Final look

Changing the appearance of a person – character make-up

When doing any character make-up, ensure you research the character thoroughly (see Chapter 5). Ensure you don't stamp your own interpretation into the make-up, unless you are instructed to do so – the general rule is to make-up the character as historically accurately as possible; collecting pictures will help you with this. The director and the actor will have very firm ideas on what the particular character should look like, and the make-up artist must interpret their ideas. Character make-up can be anything from simply adding a beard or moustache to applying make-up, postiche and prosthetics.

Male to female gender change

1 First the eyebrows were plucked to define and remove stragglers from the bridge of the nose.
2 Heavy shading was then applied to the top of the forehead, temples, cheeks, under the jaw and down the side of the neck in a mixture of brown grease and dark base grease, this was set with setting powder before the base was applied.
3 The base was set with setting powder and the collarbones were shaded and highlighted to give prominence.
4 Three eye shadow colours were applied in a manner to widen the eyes as they were quite close together.
5 The eyes were then lined using a damp brush to wet the purple eye shadow as this gives a softer look than a pencil liner.
6 Before applying dark brown mascara, a white pencil was used to line the bottom inner rim of the eye, as the eyes were quite red. This also has the effect of opening the eyes up.

EQUIPMENT AND PRODUCT LIST
Equipment and products for a man to woman make-up
Equipment
Tweezers
Foundation brush
Blusher brush
Eyeliner brush
Lip brush
Products
Grimas brown grease and dark base grease
Grimas base – to suit model's skin tone
Ben Nye eye shadows – pale lilac, mauve, dark purple
Ben Nye Warm Rose blusher
Mehron – natural lip pencil
Mehron – dark brown mascara

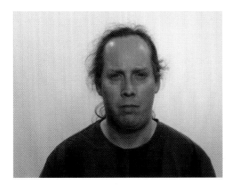

Gender reversal male to female before

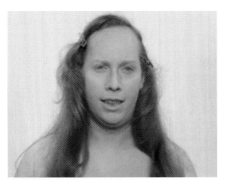

Stages 1, 2 and 3 – preparation and shading applied before setting with powder

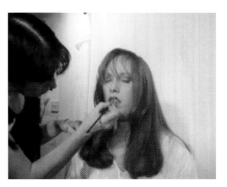

Stages 4, 5, 6 and 7 – eye and lip make-up applied, and appropriate use of blusher

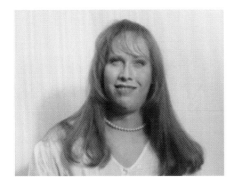

Gender reversal man to woman final

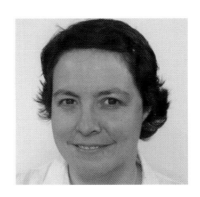

Gender reversal woman to man before

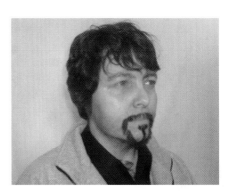

Gender reversal female to male final

7 Blusher was applied to the cheekbones, to give them prominence and the lips were lined with a natural lip pencil and filled with Clennel Calliope lipstick and finally a slick of gloss to add shine.

For instructions on gender reversing make-up from a woman to a man, see page 150.

LOOKS FROM HIT MUSICALS

Bombay Dream

This look would appear ridiculous on a Caucasian model, because the musical is set in Bombay (now known as Mumbai). The choice of model or actor is therefore important, as it makes the character more plausible.

1 Cleanse, tone and moisturise the skin.
2 To bring authenticity to this make-up, a much lighter base had to be applied and was done by using a cream foundation applied with a sponge followed by powdering with a cake make-up.

EQUIPMENT AND PRODUCT LIST
Equipment and products for Bombay Dream
Equipment
Full make-up brush set
Cleanser, toner and moisturiser
Full make-up kit
Body jewellery

3   Blusher was applied around the cheekbones, brow and hollow under chin.

4   White eye shadow was applied below the brow, followed by a butterfly wing of the turquoise. The amethyst was applied to the eye lid and blended towards the brow. Eyeliner was used by wetting a dark eye shadow and applied with a brush and mascara to separate the lashes; the eyebrows were lightly enhanced with an eyebrow pencil.

5   The lips were lined to prevent 'bleeding' and lipstick was applied with a disposable brush.

6   The look was completed with the application of body jewellery as a bindhi and props to dress the model.

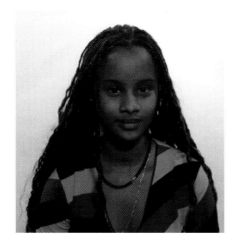

Bombay dream before

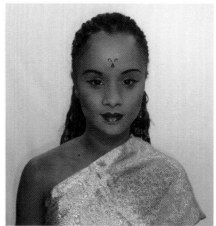

Stages 1–6 – after preparation and application of foundation, apply blusher, make up eyes and lips and apply body jewellery

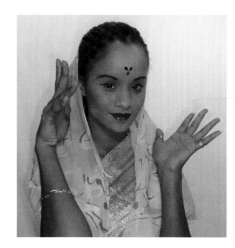

Bombay dream final look

Madam Butterfly

As with Bombay Dream, this interpretation of Madame Butterfly has been made easier by using an oriental model. If no oriental model was available, you would have to make oriental eyepieces, made with plastic or latex.

1   Cleanse, tone and moisturise the skin.

2   Apply camouflage and/or concealer to mask any skin blemishes, such as redness on cheeks and around any pustules.

3   Apply make-up base with a dampened sponge using cake make-up, blending as you go.

4   Apply blusher to cheekbones and hollow under chin.

5   Apply liquid eyeliner, asking the model to keep her eyes closed until dry.

6   Next apply beige eye shadow, blending to avoid harsh lines. Apply mascara to separate the lashes and enhance the eyebrows with an eyebrow pencil.

7   Finally, line the lips to prevent bleeding and apply lipstick using a disposable brush.

8   Dress, using props.

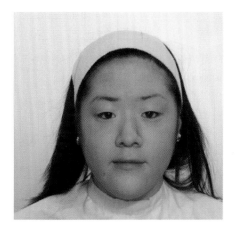

Madam Butterfly before

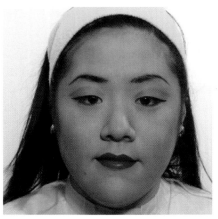

Stages 1–8 – note the difference enhancing the brows has made

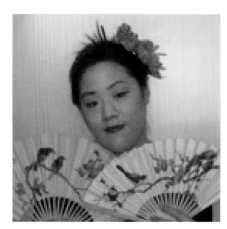

Madam Butterfly final look

Chicago

The use of appropriate props; in this case the pearls, the outfit and the hair style, all help to interpret the character to be portrayed. However, your aim should always be for the make-up alone to portray the subject. Props are of course important, but don't make the mistake of *relying* on them to portray any character.

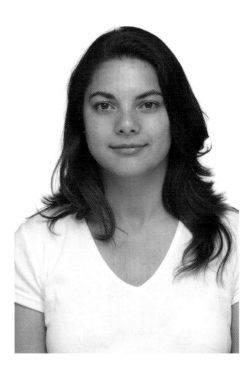

Before Chicago

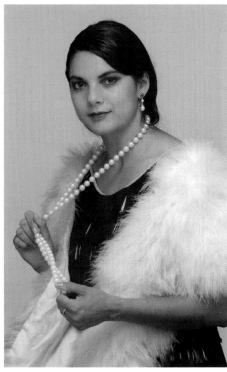

Classic make-up application of the era with good use of props

EQUIPMENT AND PRODUCT LIST
Equipment and products for Chicago
Full make-up brush set
Cleanser, toner and moisturiser
Full make-up kit
Appropriate props

Equipment and products for
Cats

Full make-up brush set

Cleanser, toner and moisturiser

Full make-up kit

Appropriate props: wigs and
whiskers

Cats

Research for this type of musical character can be done by researching on
the Internet and reading as much about the production as you can. If,
however, you get the opportunity to see any live shows, especially
productions like Cats (written by Sir Andrew Lloyd-Webber), they are
especially inspirational. Good productions are so exceptional that you
should be able to recall the images years later.

1 Cleanse and tone the skin, but do not moisturise as you have whiskers to
   stick on.
2 Camouflage make-up was used to cover skin blemishes, followed by a
   cream foundation applied with a sponge.

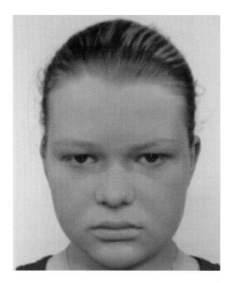

Stages 1 and 2 – prepare skin and
apply camouflage make-up

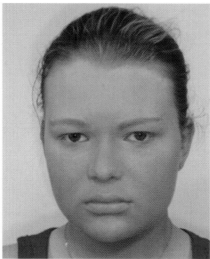

Stage 3 – apply grey face paint
starting from chin

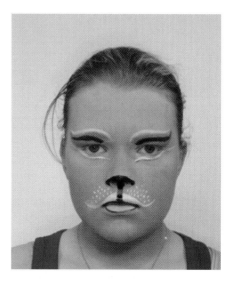

Stage 4 – apply lip and eye detail
using greasepaints

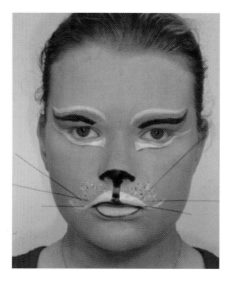

Stage 5 – fix whiskers with eyelash
adhesive

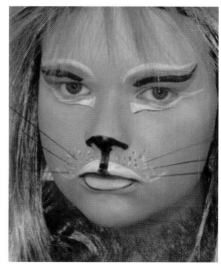

Cat look final

3 The grey was applied starting at the chin and working up so it was darkest at the chin and lightest on the cheeks.

4 Lip and eye details were applied using greasepaints and not face paints, to allow facial movement without cracking.

5 Whiskers were applied using eyelash glue, as it is a little stronger adhesive than spirit gum.

6 The wig was placed on the model's head and hair spray used to fashion the ears. Crepe hair was held against the chest and neck to finish the illusion.

CHARACTER MAKE-UP

Robin Hood and Maid Marion

With fictional or historical figures, research is important. Research the age, health and temperament of the characters and aim to portray these in your make-up.

Robin Hood

1 Cleanse and tone the skin. Do not moisturise, as the beard will not stick to the skin.

2 Veil camouflage make-up was used to cover skin blemishes, avoiding the areas of beard and moustache application.

3 Ensuring the beard and moustache areas are free from oil, apply spirit gum to these areas. Allow the spirit gum to become tacky, then firmly press the hairpieces into place. You may need to trim the lace slightly around the edges.

4 To bring authenticity to this make-up, a much lighter base had to be applied by using a cream foundation applied with a sponge followed by powdering with a cake make-up.

5 Add the light tan to the base to give the appearance of outdoor living and perhaps lack of washing.

6 Shading and highlighting were used to create facial contours.

7 A dark eye shadow was used to deepen the set of the eyes and eyebrows were lightly touched up with an eyebrow pencil.

8 The look was completed with costume and props, the hat having straightened crepe hair attached to it.

Cleaning facial hairpieces after use:

1 Ensure the room is well ventilated.

2 Lay hairpieces on a towel.

3 Using a hair colouring brush, dip into acetone, and dab at the spirit gum until removed.

4 When clean, dry the hairpieces by gently waving in the air.

5 Store in a box that is large enough not to crush them.

EQUIPMENT AND PRODUCT LIST
Equipment and products for Robin Hood
Full make-up brush set
Cleanser, toner and moisturiser
Full make-up kit
Appropriate props: pre-prepared moustache and chin beard
Spirit gum, spirit gum remover and acetone

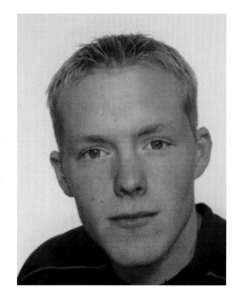

Robin Hood before

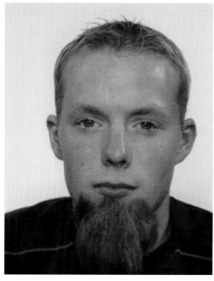

Stages 1, 2 and 3 – apply camouflage make-up. Apply spirit gum and fix hair pieces in place

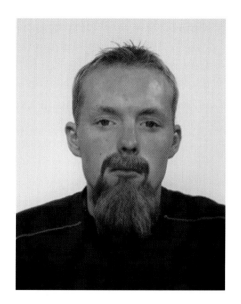

Stages 4 and 5 – work on the base adding a light tan

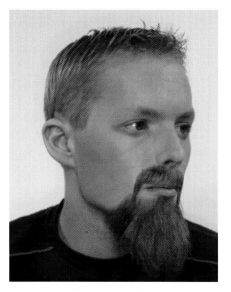

Stages 6 and 7 – apply shading and a dark shadow to deepen eyes

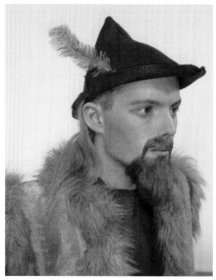

Add appropriate props to achieve the final look

EQUIPMENT AND PRODUCT LIST
Equipment and products for Maid Marion
Full make-up brush set
Cleanser, toner and moisturiser
Full make-up kit
Appropriate props

Maid Marion

1 Cleanse, tone and moisturise the skin.

2 Veil camouflage make-up was used to cover skin blemishes.

3 To bring authenticity to this make-up, a much lighter base had to be applied using a cream foundation applied with a sponge followed by powdering with a cake make-up. Shading and highlighting were used to create facial contours.

4 Highlight below the brow using a white eye shadow, eyebrows were lightly touched up with eyebrow pencil.

5   Minimal eyeliner was applied using wetted eye shadow to emphasis the eyes, and mascara, but general eye shadow was avoided as this was not a feature of the day.

6   The lips were lined to prevent 'bleeding' and the lipstick applied with a brush.

7   The look was finished off with a costume and props.

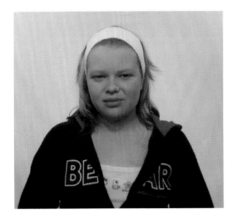

Maid Marion before

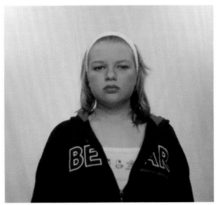

Stages 1–6 – after preparing the skin, apply camouflage base, minimal eye make-up and highlighting and contouring face

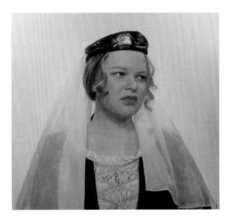

Stage 7 – add appropriate props to achieve final look – the thoughtful, romantic look of Maid Marion

Henry VIII

The choice of model is appropriate for this historical character. A skinny young man would be extremely difficult to make-up into a plausible old Henry VIII. So the choice of model or actor is again important.

1   Cleanse and tone the skin.

2   The model was chosen because of his existing beard and moustache, however some work was needed on these to start with. The beard and moustache were trimmed to tidy them up.

3   Two foundations were blended to create a fair complexion and then powdered. Shading and highlighting were used to create facial contours.

4   A red eye shadow was applied only to the edges of the eye lid and under eye area; the eyebrows were lightly enhanced with eyebrow pencil.

5   Lipstick was applied to make the lips stand out from the beard and moustache.

6   To complete the make-up, sponges were inserted into the cheek pouches to increase the roundness of the face.

7   The look was completed by the model wearing a costume of the period which included a hat.

EQUIPMENT AND PRODUCT LIST
Equipment and products for Henry VIII
Full make-up brush set
Cleanser, toner and moisturiser
Full make-up kit
Appropriate props

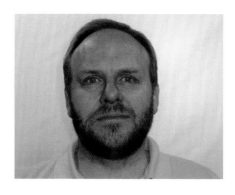

Henry VIII before

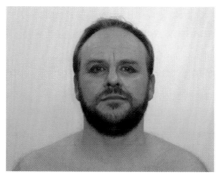

Stages 1–7 – prepare the skin, apply base and set, apply highlighting and contouring and eye and lip make-up

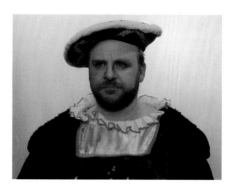

Henry VIII after

Betty Boop

Betty Boop was an American television cartoon character, and can only accurately be portrayed with black hair and arched eyebrows as this was indeed the look.

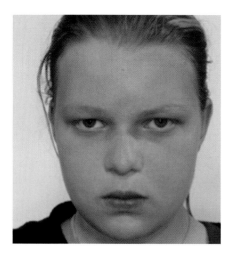

Stage 1 – apply foundation and conceal blemishes

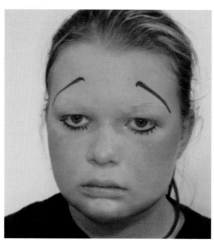

Stage 2 – block out eyebrows, paint in new 'eyebrows', lower lashes and eyebrows

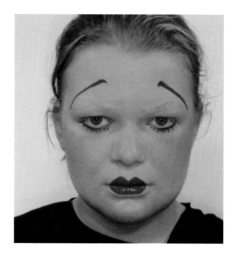

Stage 3 – shade and highlight to slim the face and apply red lipstick to emphasise the Cupid's Bow shape

EQUIPMENT AND PRODUCT LIST
Equipment and products for Betty Boop
Full make-up brush set
Cleanser, toner and moisturiser
Full make-up kit
Eyebrow wax for blocking out
Wigs and earrings

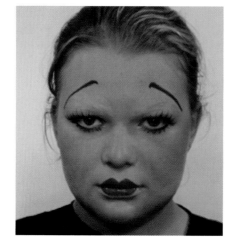

Stage 4 – apply false lashes to top lashes

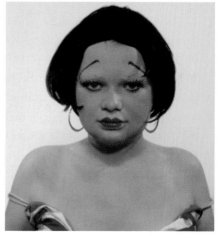

Stage 5 – complete by adding appropriate wig and earrings for final look

MAKE-UP ARTIST PROFILE: PIPPA HAYNE

Pippa Hayne is Head of Department for Beauty, Hair & Holistic Therapies at Totton College, Hampshire. She is a qualified hairdresser, nail technician, beauty therapist, holistic therapist, sports therapist and make-up artist. She is able to teach all of the subjects as well as carry them out into the commercial world.

How and when did you start in the business?

I underwent a complete career change at the age of thirty, through initially having an interest in hairdressing. I gained the qualification and haven't stopped acquiring new skills since.

Was there a turning point in your career?

I think the turning point for me was carrying out make-up on my daughter to match the character for fancy dress parties and finding I was rather good at it. This led me to begin my career in beauty, which in turn led me to pursue qualifications and work in theatrical and media make-up.

What do you consider to be important qualities for a make-up artist?

Good research skills, adaptability, imagination, able to work under pressure, a team player but also able to work alone if needs be. But most of all to enjoy what you are doing.

What is your most memorable/exciting/best paid job?

My most memorable job was carrying out the make-up for a large group of under privileged youngsters who were appearing in a dance show production. The production had been organised to bring these talented kids to the attention of producers and choreographers in the business. The memorable outcome was that many of them were offered opportunities to begin a career in the industry.

Have you had any disasters?

We all have disasters, however, I learnt very early on to practise whatever I was doing before the big day and not leave things to chance – as that is usually when they go very wrong.

What advice would you give to young people entering the industry?

I would suggest they gain a basic make-up and hairdressing qualification, and then go on to a theatrical and media make-up qualification. By this time they would be over eighteen and allowed to work in the media, television and film industry. It is also a good idea, whilst training, to attach yourself to an amateur dramatics society and do all the make-up and hair for their productions. This way you will really know if you enjoy it and can take the pressure involved.

In your experience, would you advise those training to become make-up artists to specialise in one area only, or to gain experience, through Continued Professional Development courses (CPD) in many different areas of make-up?

I would suggest that initially a basic qualification be gained, spend a little time using it gaining experience, and then start to attend a few workshops introducing yourself to new and different skills. Have a go at these new skills before deciding if you really want to offer them and then if you do, sign up for a full-blown qualification.

Clear instructions – make sure you understand what is required of you

Pantomime vs. fashion: fresh and freckles

These fresh and freckles looks give a good example of the differences between theatrical make-up and fashion make-up. Theatrical 'freckles' make-up should be bold, bright and fun and should be seen from a distance, whereas a fashion 'freckles' make-up is precise and delicate. The freckles must be seen in each look, one significantly so and one realistically so. With the theatrical freckles the face has been made up strongly and cleanly. Strongly because both the strength of the light and the distance will reduce the impact of the make-up (the freckles), and cleanly because otherwise the facial definition will fail to register at a distance.

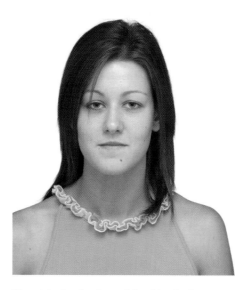

Theatrical – fresh and freckles before

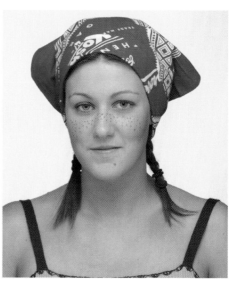

Theatrical – fresh and freckles after

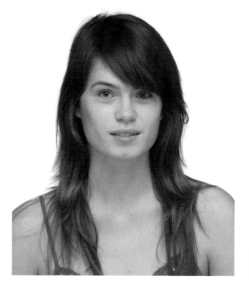

Fashion – fresh and freckles before

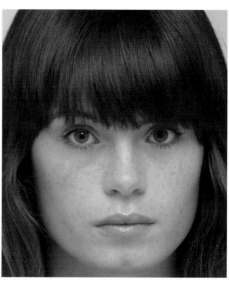

Fashion – fresh and freckles after

With the fashion freckles, the make-up has been applied precisely and delicately. Precisely because the camera will pick up every brush stroke, and therefore every freckle, and delicately because the brief was a 'fresh and freckles' look. The camera will pick up on these 'make-up' freckles so they need to look 'real' – not theatrical. Both looks are correct for their intended purpose.

EYES FOR SPECIAL EFFECTS

Contact lenses can provide anything from a subtle eye colour change to extremely dramatic effects. They can be bought 'off the shelf' but, because these may be dangerous to the eyes of the wearer, having lenses made to measure is recommended, especially if they are to enhance a specific character. Choose companies who have their own team of contact lens technicians and who specialise in special effects contact lenses for film, TV and media industries. These companies have hundreds of lenses, including eyes resembling blindness, blood filled, alien, and every conceivable colour. Lenses are sometimes hand painted or can be tinted or stamped, according to the budget available. All the company will ask for is a concept of the character – who they are, the role they are going to play and what they are going to look like as the character. It is usually the responsibility of the assistant make-up artist to look after the lenses, to clean them and to stand by the actor at all times to check they are worn only for the recommended safety time under health and safety regulations and the optician's recommendations. The assistant make-up artist will accompany the actor in case there is a problem with the lenses.

HEALTH AND SAFETY

Never use the same set of lenses on different actors – this is against all normal hygiene practices.

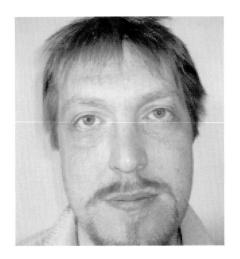

Model with own coloured eyes

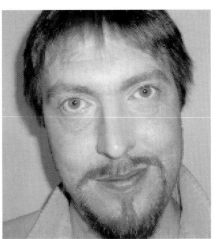

Model with 'green' eyes

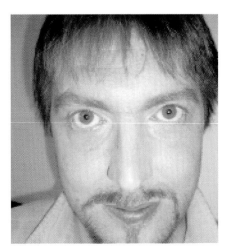

Model with 'blue' eyes

BALD CAPS

Making a bald cap on a head block

Bald caps are specifically made plastic caps intended to simulate a bald head. In television and film work, this is often a key factor in making a character look older. Ready made bald caps are usually used, however it is interesting to know how to make your own – which can be very cost effective, as ready-made caps tend to be expensive.

To make a plastic bald cap you will need a head block, which needs to be prepared before any product is used. Sometimes when head blocks are new, the centre join line needs to be filed down and smoothed out. You prepare the block by smearing over it a very thin coat of Vaseline, and wiping it over with a tissue. You can then apply the plastic following the manufacturer's instructions. Bald cap plastic usually comes in liquid form and comprises PVC and PVA and a plasticiser. Painting layers of the liquid plastic onto the solid head block makes the cap. Each layer of plastic will take about ten minutes to dry – depending upon the product being used. Do not apply the next coat until the previous one is completely dry.

For a good fit plastic bald cap, you can make a pattern out of cling film. The cling film is wrapped around the head, secured with adhesive tape. With a marker pen, draw the hairline and the ears over the cling film. By making a small cut in the cling film (over the ear is a good place), the cling film pattern can be removed from the model's head. Carefully cut around the marked outline of the hairline, and the pattern can then be placed on the head block. With a pencil, draw around the pattern, slightly larger than it is. Remove the cling film pattern and discard. With the head block prepared apply layers of liquid plastic with a medium sized paintbrush. The paintbrush will have to be cleaned with **acetone** in between each layer of plastic. Be methodical in your application, work from the top to the edges, keeping each layer as thin as possible. Depending upon the product being used, you may need up to eight layers before the cap is finished. To remove

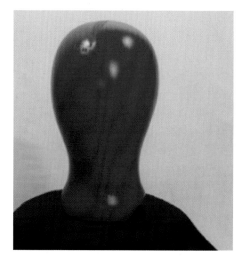

Head block

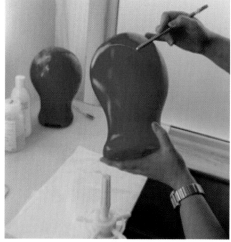

Marking the hairline with a white marker

the bald cap from the block, a T-pin and a powdered puff is used to gently ease the plastic cap away from the head block.

Making the pattern will give you good measurements around the hairline and over the ears, but the size will be determined by the size of head block you have – usually just a standard size. If you have no time to make a plastic pattern, you can, especially with practice, just make your outline directly onto the head block. Using a white marker, mark the hairline and ear positions, and proceed according to the manufacturer's instructions.

Step by step bald cap

Applying the bald cap:

1 Before application of a bald cap, prepare the hair by combing short hair as flat as possible or by wrapping long hair and placing a stocking cap on top to keep hair secure. Try to use as few hair grips as possible and position them so they won't be visible or likely to tear the bald cap.

2 Place the bald cap on to the head carefully checking the position to ensure it covers the hairline. Once smoothed out, carefully cut the bald cap along the hairline leaving a 2 cm gap between the edge and the hairline. When cutting the cap around the ears ensure the cut is precise enough to not crease the cap or misshape the ear when the cap is pulled tight.

3 If the bald cap is made from latex rubber, ensure the cut line is slightly wavy to help disguise the joins later. If the cap is made from cap plastic then cutting a wavy line is unnecessary, as the edge will be melted away with the use of acetone.

4 To glue the cap, start at the front by applying spirit gum to the under edge of the cap on the forehead section up to the temples, wait for the spirit gum to go tacky, and then place down on to the skin and remove any air bubbles by pushing out towards the edges.

5 Glue the section of the cap at the centre back of the neck (nape). Ask the model to slightly lift their head and this will help to tighten the bald cap when the head is in the normal position.

6 Glue the temple areas of the cap up to the front of the ears, pull the cap downwards and forwards to increase the tension and ensure the cap stays smooth. Finally, glue the sides at the back of the neck by pulling downwards and towards the front to once again increase the tension of the cap.

7 If the cap is latex rubber, the next step is similar to disguising the joins of a latex prosthetic piece, that is applying layers of liquid latex by stippling over the edge of the cap onto the skin. Wait for the latex to dry before adding another layer. Apply as many layers as needed to disguise the edge of the cap.

8 If the cap is made from cap plastic, pour some acetone into a glass jar and, with a cotton wool bud, apply the acetone onto the edge of the cap using a sidewards rubbing motion. After a couple of seconds the bald cap starts to melt and you can smooth the edge of the cap with a final downward movement with the cotton bud.

HEALTH AND SAFETY

Regularly change the cotton bud as it gets saturated in melted plastic. As you are using acetone, be extremely careful when working anywhere in the facial areas, and particularly careful when working above the eye area.

TIP

It is recommended not to moisturise the skin if you are applying postiche, as the adhesive will have difficulty in adhering to the moisturised skin.

Applying make-up to a bald cap

1 The white and flesh base was applied with a large flat brush to create smooth, straight lines.
2 Black outlining and detail was applied with a medium flat brush and blended pinks were stippled with a dry latex sponge.
3 The whole make-up was fixed with a neutral powder. However, a white powder can be used in these circumstances to give a brilliant white effect to the base.
4 The large red sponge nose was added to finish.

EQUIPMENT AND PRODUCT LIST

Equipment and products for bald cap

Paradise Aqua colours

Powders – neutral and white

Large red sponge

Selection of make-up brushes

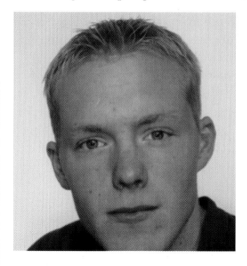
Before clown

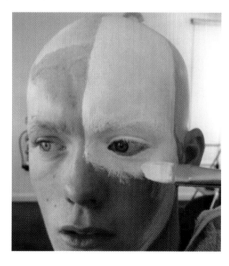
Stage 1 – apply base with large brush

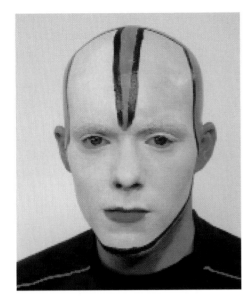

Stage 2 – add black and red detail with a medium flat brush

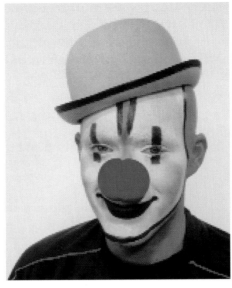

Stages 2, 3 and 4 – stipple pink colour to selected areas and fix with white powder. Add nose and hat to create final result

You don't always need to buy or make a bald cap as indicated by our model emulating a character from the Addams Family!

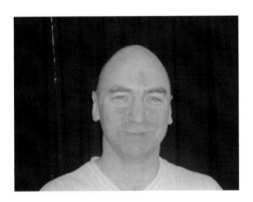

Addams Family before

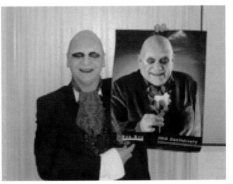

Addams Family after

PROSTHETICS

Custom made prosthetics

Custom made prosthetics are 3D (three dimensional) pieces designed to alter the shape of a face or body for use in theatre and television, usually for horror or fantasy effects, but also for character changing work. Examples include false ears, eye bags, swollen eye pieces, chins and noses. They are normally made of latex or plastic and can be fixed in position with spirit gum or other suitable adhesives. The edges are sealed and blended with latex and are painted with greasepaint or camouflage make-up to blend in with the rest of the design. Prosthetics are available from professional make-up suppliers and are suitable for use in theatre, film and TV. Prosthetics must always be attached to the skin according to the manufacturer's instructions.

Step by step instructions for Werewolf

1 Ensure the face is cleansed and toned, but not moisturised as the postiche will not stick.

2 Block out the eyebrows.

3 Check that the pre-bought prosthetic pieces fit the model correctly before application.

4 Apply a heavy layer of red toned blusher powder to the prosthetic pieces; this acts as the blood supply to the false pieces. Once the skin tone is applied, it is not seen but it prevents the pieces looking chalky and false.

5 Apply the skin tone onto the pieces in the form of greasepaint cream foundations or rubber mask grease.

6 Mark the outline of the prosthetic onto the face with a little powder on a powder puff.

7 Apply prosthetic adhesive following the outline of the piece only. Most prosthetic pieces have a frilly edge, which is thinner than the rest of the piece, this identifies the area to be glued and helps to make the joins easier to disguise.

8 Once the prosthetic adhesive is a little tacky, apply the piece and press down the edges firmly, check the position to ensure it is straight.

9 Next, using the same prosthetic adhesive, stipple the joins of the pieces onto the real skin in thin layers, to help disguise the edges.

10 Once the pieces are on, proceed with applying greasepaint or cream foundation, in the same colour of skin tone as used on the pieces, to the rest of the face using a dry latex sponge. The greasepaint or cream foundation should be the same colour for the real skin.

11 Appropriate highlighting, shading and detailing are applied to the skin, prosthetic pieces and blocked brows with greasepaint or cream foundations.

12 Once all greasepaint products have been applied, apply powder to fix.

13 On all the areas requiring facial hair, apply a layer of spirit gum onto the skin in the appropriate area, slightly larger than the shape of the cut crepe hair. Once tacky, hold the crepe hair at the correct angle and, with the hand close to the cut edges, place the ends onto the adhesive without folding them over. The effect should look like the crepe hair is actually growing directly from the skin.

14 Continue to do this on all areas requiring facial hair, remembering to adjust the angle so it is growing 45 degrees (perpendicular) to the face.

15 Finally gently comb/dress the crepe hair by using the tail of a tail comb, pulling through the hair. Don't be surprised by the quantity of hair which may come out, as long as the effect isn't left bald, you will have correctly glued the hair and left the spirit gum to dry.

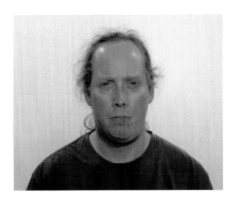

Werewolf before

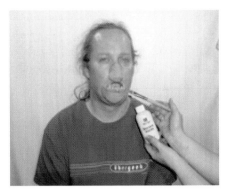

Stages 1–9 – prepare skin and eyebrows and apply prosthetic pieces

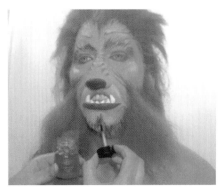

Stage 10–12 – apply base and highlights. Shade in appropriate areas and powder to fix

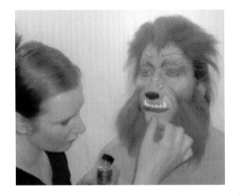

Stage 13 – apply spirit gum to areas requiring facial hair

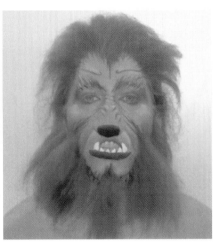

Comb and dress crepe hair

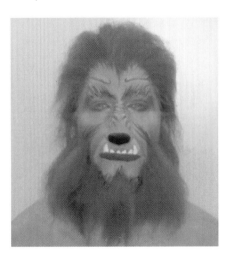

Werewolf – final

How prosthetics are made

If a ready made prosthetic is unsuitable for a particular character, prosthetics can be individually made to match an actor's face or body part. These made-to-measure pieces, or appliances, are made in a flexible material such as plastic, rubber or gelatine, and can be applied to the actor's face or body, giving a perfect fit. Full **life casting** is not a requirement of an NVQ theatrical and media qualification, but is something you will learn if you proceed to specialise in theatrical make-up. However, as an introduction to making prosthetics, and to some of the materials used, an example is given here making small prosthetic pieces for a Halloween character.

Designing your own characters – making small prosthetic pieces

Designing a character from scratch gives you a fantastic opportunity to use your imagination. The example here shows how a Halloween character has been designed and created and includes new techniques and tips that will help you create your own characters. As the prosthesis is relatively small, a life cast of the actor is not required, so the model can be created on a tile or piece of glass.

TIP	

A life cast is a prosthetics piece that is made to measure for an individual model. First a mask is made to match the model and, from this, a duplicate positive casting is made with a material such as plaster or stone: this is called a face cast or body cast. From this a new shape is sculpted and is called a 'positive'.

| TIP | |

Whenever you get the opportunity to use your imagination, use it! It will help you to stand out from the crowd.

| TIP | |

Smaller prostheses modelling for the face can be created on one of those full size glass heads that are sold as ornaments. It will save you a lot of money in life cast materials. They are also very good for making bald caps on.

| TIP | |

A good quality water-based clay is best for prosthetics modelling. It must be kept wet and sealed inside a plastic bag.

EQUIPMENT AND PRODUCT LIST

Equipment and products for a Halloween character

Equipment

Gown for client

Plastic box

Tile or piece of glass

Modelling knife

Sand paper

Wooden waxing spatula

Old latex sponge

Hair dryer (optional)

Scissors

Hair spray

Measure

Products

Modelling clay

Plaster

Round balsa wood

Liquid latex

Translucent powder

Eyeliner pencil

Spirit gum

Aqua colours paints and powders

Grimas 'Old Age' colour

Blood (optional)

Pre-bought crepe hair

DONFAB   FABULOUS FX

PRODUCTION:

Base __OA (OLD AGE)__

Highlight _____

Shading __DARK BROWN POWDER__

Powder _____

Moist rouge _____

Dry rouge _____

Lip colour _____

EYE MAKE-UP:

Shadow __DARK BROWN POWDER__

Highlight _____

Pencil _____

Eye lines __RED UNDER EYES ONLY__

Mascara _____

False lashes _____

Lip colour __BLACK__

Body make-up _____

ADDITIONAL DETAILS __LATEX PROSTHESES TO BE FITTED BEFORE BASE. EYEBROWS TO BE PAINTED ON WITH AQUA (BLACK). GREY CREPE HAIR FOR BEARD. FIXED WITH SPIRIT GUM.__

MAKE-UP ARTIST PROFILE: ANDY DONLEY

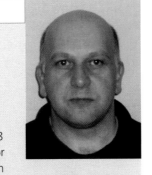

Andy Donley is a make-up artist, visiting college lecturer and supplier of theatrical make-up.

How and when did you start in the business?

Well, I was a late starter as they say! I had been quite happy working at my chosen career as a toolmaker (engineer) for 18 years or so. Then it happened, a friend asked me to model for them at college. That was the first time I had been involved in theatrical make-up. Within the week I was asked if I wanted to have a look backstage at our local theatre. That turned out to be a trick as the make-up crew were short handed and needed someone gullible to help. The next thing I knew I was back to modelling, this time for a casualty exercise for the fire service, great fun, lots of prosthetics and I was hooked. So it was off to college to gain some qualifications of my own. All that only happened within the last eight years.

Was there a turning point in your career?

Well I don't think I had a turning point, but a total career change. I did become a lot more focused (my wife would say obsessed) when I was fortunate enough to win a couple of national make-up awards. This was fun as it did then lead onto a small TV appearance as the engineer who became a make-up artist. Although I have been asked if I would like to work in TV or film, my love is in the theatre. That being said, I have been known to make a few bits and pieces for TV adverts and film.

What do you consider to be important qualities for a make-up artist?

First and foremost I think you have to be dedicated, as there are usually a lot of people depending on you. You must keep up to date with new products and methods, there is so much happening out there and you need to be a part of it if you want to stay ahead of the rest.

What is your most memorable/exciting/best paid job?

The most memorable job was one with two hundred dancers for us to make-up, with an added challenge of producing all the stage special effects as well. The make-up went well, but everything that could go wrong with the special effects did. From a cherry picker [lift] turning into a metronome at about fifteen feet off the ground (this would have been funny if it wasn't for the fact that I was the one on it), to pyrotechnics detonating themselves (that makes you jump!). The thing to note here is that the show was a tremendous success.

The most exciting job is always the next job, as you don't know what it is going to be!

The best paid job – any job that you have enjoyed working on and been paid for has got to be the best paid job!

Have you had any disasters?

Of course I have, but one that jumps into my head is when I was involved with dancing skeletons. Their costumes were painted with UV reactive paint and they wore UV reactive masks. On stage they were lit up with a UV cannon, and it looked fantastic. That is until I decided to try out this new make-up that I had found that was also UV reactive. I thought I would remove one mask and replace it with this new make-up. GOOD IDEA! NO! the dancers came on stage and one was somewhat noticeable – as he didn't have a head!!

What advice would you give to young people entering the industry?

Get as much training as you can, try everything, and then learn the job from people who are already doing it. I have found that this is a great industry to be involved in because we all tend to help each other and we are all still learning ourselves. I almost forgot to say IT'S FUN.

In your experience, would you advise those training to become make-up artists to specialise in one area only, or to gain experience, through Continued Professional Development courses (CPD) in many different areas of make-up?

Yes, gain as much experience through CPD in as many different areas as possible, then you can choose which way you want to go.

TIP

When laying out your make-up brushes, it is a good idea to put them in a container all pointing straight up. When you use one, place it on the worktop facing down. This way you can see at a glance which brushes are clean and which ones are unused.

The first thing to think about with this Halloween character is the exit wounds for the horns. These will be sculptured out of modelling clay and made to the exact shape required. When you are completely happy with your models, you will need to measure the diameter of the holes in the centre, as these will have to have horns made to fit into them. Carefully remove them from the tile or piece of glass and place them into a suitable plastic box – one that will allow you to cast the model prosthesis. You can also build a wall of clay around it for protection.

Making the plaster cast

After mixing the plaster with water, according to the manufacturer's instructions, scoop out a small amount of plaster from the mixing bowl and gently pour it over the models, making sure that it gets into all the little nooks and crannies. Also make sure you don't create any bubbles on the surface of the models, as these will create cavities in your finished mould. Now fill the mould with the rest of the plaster. Tap it gently to release any air bubbles. After you have filled your mould leave it to set, according to the manufacturer's instructions.

Take a length of round balsa wood the same diameter or bigger than your prosthetic cavity. Carve a horn shape at one end of a full length of balsa – it will be cut to length later. After the basic shape has been made, sand off any blemishes or sharp angles to form the finished horn, and cut to length. Repeat the process to create the second horn. Once the mould has set, tip it out of its box or remove the clay wall you made to contain the plaster. The modelling clay must now be removed from the new negative mould. Don't use sharp objects as you will carve new unwanted features into the mould walls. Most clay will just pull out with your fingers and the rest can be worked out with part of a wooden waxing spatula.

TIP

Plaster of Paris is a soft plaster and dental stone is a hard plaster. Plaster moulds are usually reinforced with fibres or fabrics such as scrim, sacking, hessian or horsehair.

TIP

Balsa wood is a versatile material to use in the creation of prosthetics. It is very light so it will not pull the creation off. It looks as good as bone, horn or even steel if you spray it. It can be carved, sanded, glued and painted.

Moulding the prosthetic

The mould is now ready to be filled with liquid latex. Dab around the top edge of the mould with an old latex sponge and let it air dry.

The mould can be left to set overnight, which is recommended, but you can speed things up considerably with the aid of a hairdryer. Alternatively leave the mould near to a radiator, making sure you have plenty of ventilation.

To remove the prosthetic from the mould, first dust the surface with translucent powder. This will stop the latex sticking to itself while you are removing it from the mould. Gently grab the edge of the prosthetic (you may have to roll the edge up with your finger before you can find anything to pull on). Now just gently pull it out of the mould. Dust it off with translucent powder and place it in an airtight container until it is needed. Give the mould a little dusting of powder and refill with latex. It is always a good idea to make a few spares, as you will only use these prosthetics once.

> **TIP**
>
> If you want to create a much larger prosthetic without the expense of using foam latex, then try getting hold of a *new* latex foam cushion available from most markets. Cut and shape it with an electric calving knife then coat it in liquid latex to form a barrier between the inferior industrial quality latex and your client's skin. This will also help to remove any blemishes in your sculpture. Take great care when using knives.

> **HEALTH AND SAFETY** ✚
>
> Never be tempted to use the cheaper industrial quality liquid latex that is available as modelling latex. It is too poor a grade of latex and is not suitable to be put onto skin. People can develop an allergic reaction to any grade of latex at any time.

> **TIP** ✔
>
> You should find it difficult to find the edges of a well fitted prosthetic and dabbing around the edge of the mould after filling with latex will give you a very thin edge to the prosthetic, making it easier to loose the edge when fitting it to the model.

> **HEALTH AND SAFETY** ✚
>
> Always read and adhere to manufacturer's instructions on all products you use.

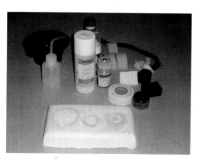

Work set up area with prosthetics

The preparation work has been completed for our Halloween character. We have two exit wounds and two horns. We can begin to create our character.

1 Prepare the work area before the model arrives – this will allow you to make a visual check that you have everything you need.

> **TIP** ✔
>
> Spirit gum can get messy, so either use latex gloves or have a cleansing pad dusted in translucent powder so that if you manage to get spirit gum on your fingers, you can just dab your fingers onto the pad and this will stop you sticking to your client.

2 Cover the model with a protective gown and seat comfortably. Decide on the positioning of prosthetic exit wounds. Once you have decided, mark the areas with an eyeliner pencil.

3 Coat the back of one of the prosthetics with spirit gum and place it onto the pre-marked position. Lift it away and replace it a few times until you see strings of gum forming between prosthetic and client. It will now stick well without sliding on the skin.

> **TIP**
>
> Try the prosthetic on the client before gluing it, and if it needs trimming don't cut it down with scissors, tear it! A straight cut will always show up as a line on your finished work.

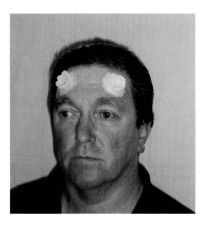

Fitted prosthetics

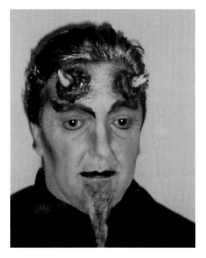

Completed Halloween character

4 Press down the edges of the prosthetic – this is where those very thin edges come into their own – once you are happy and all the edges are stuck down, dab all around the edges with latex milk with an old latex sponge. This should help you to lose those edges altogether. Apply the other prosthetic in the same way.

5 Using aqua colours, you can now make-up the model. A change in skin colour around the protruding horns would be expected as they have 'broken through the skin'. Using the colour OA (old age), apply, starting at the top of the model's face and working down. When working around the prosthetics, stipple the colour on (don't colour inside the cavity of the prosthetic). This will give you a much bolder colour and you won't be wiping the make-up off with the sponge. Refer to your original worksheets and make-up plan, to apply shadows. Apply shadows and highlights with aqua powders using the appropriate brushes. Add all other colours according to your worksheet, which will only leave the horns and crepe hair to be applied.

6 The horns can be applied into the cavities in the prosthetics with spirit gum. If you find that the horns are slightly too small in diameter, don't worry, as you can fill the gap with scratch blood or Vaseline coloured with stage blood.

7 Prepare the crepe hair according to the make-up plan – by mixing two colours together. Once the mixing is complete, start to fit the layered beard (see Chapter 10). Three lengths of hair are required. Don't worry if it is too long at this stage, it can be trimmed later. The first layer will be applied with spirit gum to the point of the chin, the second behind and the third in front. Once fitted, trim to shape and spray with a strong hold hair spray.

TIP	

If you were to need this type of beard for a number of shows, you could paint latex onto the chin of the glass head. Give the area of chin that requires the beard a few coats and then construct your beard onto that. Use the latex rather than spirit gum to apply the hair, and when finished, gently remove and powder the latex part of it. Apply a strip or two of toupee tape and you have a reusable crepe hair beard.

Assessment of knowledge and understanding

Knowledge review

1 What product is most often used in wound make-up?

2 Why would you want to block out eyebrows?

3 If eyebrow wax were not available, what else could you use?

4 Other than eyebrows, what areas can be blocked out with wax?

5 What six colours are in the bruise colour wheel?

6 Before creating a bullet wound, what in particular would you need to research?

7 What are the two principal techniques of ageing?

8 What is the purpose of shading?

9 What is the purpose of highlighting?

10 What are bald caps used for?

11 Give four examples of custom made prosthetics.

12 What are prosthetics made from?

13 What is a life cast?

14 What is the best way to work with clay?

15 What are the advantages of working with balsa wood?

16 What is the difference between rigid and flexible Collodion?

17 Where are you most likely to encounter a graze?

18 How would you make a 'grit' effect?

19 What is meant by the term character make-up?

20 What are you trying to find out when researching historical or fictional characters?

chapter 12

Camouflage make-up

Camouflage make-up is used to cover pigmentation and other skin disorders, which are caused either by irregularities in the skin's melanin production or as a result of burning or surgery. These skin disorders are not infectious and are not contra indicated to make-up application. Camouflage make-up incorporates a large range of work including the covering of tattoos, burns or scars or teaching a daily make-up routine for someone with a visible facial birthmark. Camouflage make-up artists will also meet men, women and children who have undergone surgery for cancer or burns and need guidance in the correct use of camouflage make-up. It is because of this type of work that camouflage make-up artists are special people. They are kind, patient, tactful, sympathetic and professional. In the first instance, knowledge of corrective and fashion make-up is a great advantage to camouflage make-up artists, as they can then also advise on other make-up techniques.

Learning objectives

In this chapter you will learn about:

- **camouflage make-up products**
- **scars**
- **port wine stains and other birthmarks**
- **tattoos**
- **vitiligo**
- **chloasma**

CAMOUFLAGE MAKE-UP PRODUCTS

Camouflage products differ from ordinary cosmetics in the following ways:

- they have greater covering qualities
- they have better holding power, and are designed to stay in place longer

- they are resistant to the harmful rays of the sun
- they are waterproof
- they come in a greater variety of colours for all ethnic skin tones.

There are many excellent ranges of camouflage make-up, several of which can be obtained through the National Health Service. The two in our photograph are Covermark, USA and Dermablend Corrective Cosmetics.

Covermark, USA

Covermark produce a range of camouflage creams and powders that are used in hospitals and clinics. They are quite heavy in texture, thereby having good coverage. They have a large range of colours, which can be mixed together to obtain the exact shade of colour required.

Dermablend Corrective Cosmetics

Dermablend also has a vast range of colours, ranging from ivory to the darkest ebony, and being a corrective make-up, also has excellent coverage. Whilst suitable for all skin tones, they are particularly useful for the warm golden browns necessary for dark skins.

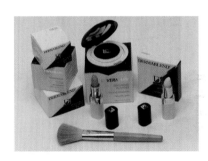

Camouflage make-up products

There are of course many other products available for corrective camouflage make-up. One suitable for make-up artists working in film, TV, fashion and theatre is Veil by Thomas Blake. This is a British company and as well as being an excellent product with many colours, it is also very cost effective. Dermacolour produced by Kryolan, and Keromask are also recommended as being very good products for camouflage make-up.

The most important aspect of camouflage make-up is the ability to choose the correct colour to cover the imperfection. If the colour chosen is too light it will look unnatural and pale, making the products obvious, whereas if the colour is too dark, it will look fake. There are colour charts available with most brands of camouflage make-up and it is a good idea to recommend that clients have a range of colours for the changing seasons. It is usual for clients to wear a lighter colour in the winter months and a darker and warmer colour in the summer months to compliment the natural change in skin colour with the sun. Camouflage make-up is usually thicker than standard foundations, and is usually applied in layers, until the imperfection is covered.

TIP
Apply camouflage make-up in natural daylight whenever possible, as it gives a better finish.

All companies providing camouflage-covering creams also produce loose powder for setting the foundation cover. The powders are nearly always translucent, being of no colour, and therefore not affecting the perfect colour of cover foundation you have chosen or mixed for the client. The ranges also have blushers to complement the colour of cover bought.

TIP
If several shades of camouflage cream are needed to match skin colour, offer to mix the shade for the client and re-pot it for them.

PREPARATION OF THE SKIN

Preparing the area of skin that requires concealer is very important. The area needs to be cleansed free of grease, dirt and make-up and then toned. Facial skin will need to be moisturised. If the skin is combination or oily, the need for anti-shine control is important because, as the day progresses, the shine will come through the make-up and leave a slightly tacky feeling. It is recommended that regular touching up be done, using either a powder from the same range as the covering cream or a translucent (colourless) powder. This will keep the make-up completely set and will take on the colour of the covering cream being used.

SOME BASIC CAMOUFLAGE TECHNIQUES

Simple scars

To many people, having a scar may not be a problem, but to others it may be quite traumatic, as they may see it as disfiguring. Scars may appear more noticeable at certain times: when going out somewhere or whilst on holiday, as less clothes may be worn and a scar that is usually covered may be uncovered for a few hours or for a few weeks. The photos show a simple leg scar before and after the application of camouflage make-up.

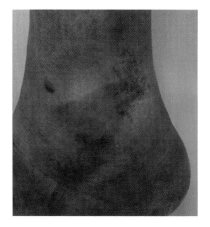

Before ankle

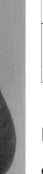

After camouflage

TIP	✔
Take your time in selecting the correct camouflage colour. In camouflage make-up the choice of colour is as important as its application.	

Broken capillaries

General camouflage make-up can be offered to men and women who have broken capillaries anywhere on the body. Generally these are covered by make-up only when they are on the face, but they can also be covered if required anywhere else on the body.

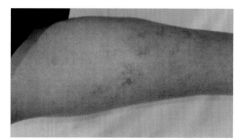

Broken capillaries before

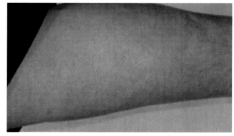

Broken capillaries after camouflage make-up

MAKE-UP ARTIST PROFILE: DONNA JONES

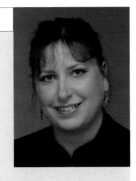

How and when did you start in the business?

I qualified in beauty therapy in June 2004 from Coleg Menai College in Bangor, North Wales and am currently undertaking further studies in beauty therapy, holistic therapies and camouflage make-up. I am qualified in Indian Head Massage and am a British Association of Skin Camouflage member.

Was there a turning point in your career?

I had decided from a very early age to help and support people with skin discolouration and disfigurements. Growing up with a port wine stain, I felt the need to pass on my experience to enable clients to feel confident in the use of camouflage products and to show the results that can be achieved.

What do you consider to be important qualities for a make-up artist?

In my situation, you require experience using the different selections of camouflage products available, knowing the techniques of blending, for that complete natural look, which is the aim of any concealment! Having *compassion* for people that are distressed and lack confidence but having the *passion* to please, give hope and successfully transform their look into something positive!

What is your most memorable/exciting/best paid job?

Being able to help with the camouflage section of this book was a very memorable time for me. It gave me the opportunity to gain confidence in exposing the 'real me', as being 'make-up free' always made me feel vulnerable. Now it has pushed me forward and given me the passion and insight I needed in order to further my career in camouflage make-up. I know by doing this I will help people in a similar situation to me, gain the knowledge, tips and confidence needed to lead their life the way they want – and fit in!

Have you had any disasters?

No disasters yet! – I guess there will be one lurking around the corner though!

What advice would you give to young people entering the industry?

Go for it! It's hard work, completely underrated and underpaid but if you enjoy working with all different types of people and get a real buzz from turning bodies and faces around into something wonderful, follow your heart and go!

Port wine stain

A port wine stain is a flat, pink, red, or purplish lesion (area of tissue with impaired function as a result of physical damage by disease or wounding), in this instance caused by blood vessel abnormality, capillary malformation of the skin. Port wine stains are usually on the face, but with correct camouflage make-up, they can be totally covered up.

How to cover a facial birth mark

This section was written by Donna Jones – model and camouflage make-up artist.

1 Wash your hands and prepare the area to be camouflaged.

2 Using a clean spatula (which comes with most products), take a small amount of product and, with a clean index or ring finger, warm the cream on the spatula in circular movements to give a workable consistency, making the product easier to apply.

3 Apply the cream in a dabbing/patting motion which won't pull at the skin, bearing in mind that you should be working with a little of the product at a time (less is more); gradually work up to more colour/more coverage. Your aim is to make this look as natural as possible. This make-up is noticeably thicker than other foundations/concealers, and so it is important not to layer it too thickly.

4 Blending is the most important part of the application, as you need the make-up to sit on the skin as naturally as possible and not to be recognised as just covering a particular blemish or disfigurement. Take the cream lightly around the area, in a thinner spread, paying more attention to the edge of the blemish and normal skin tone. The need to blend in this area is crucial for the make-up to look its best.

5 As this make-up is a concealing tool, utilise it to cover up any spots, under eye darkness, broken capillaries, etc. When making myself up, I take the cream right up to the eye and have complete coverage of any dark circles and shadows. The nose is a little tricky, as you can miss blending correctly around the nostrils and the sides are sometimes out of view. Take your time to go over the whole area, after you have finished, to touch-up or re-blend any little areas. Another helpful hint is to remember the downy hair some models have, which becomes more noticeable when you have applied make-up. Go over gently in the direction of hair growth, which will make the cream covering less obvious. A make-up wedge is useful for this job.

6 Working around the mouth can be a little difficult, especially if you need to make the actual lip line. Take the cream right around the lip, concealing and blending. If you happen to allow the cream to impose on the lip area, don't worry, sometimes it is better to wipe away excess after the setting powder has been applied, this way you get a more even look to the area. Lip liner can be added as part of the make-up routine.

7 In the same way as any other foundation, you will need to ensure that the neck area is blended in well. The nightmare of someone noticing that they can see a tidemark is embarrassing and makes the make-up less natural. Take the make-up as far down as necessary to achieve the blending process correctly.

8 Setting powder. When you are satisfied with the cream application, the make-up can be set, using setting powder. These generally come with a powder puff. I find the thick, fluffy variety easier to use, although you can waste a lot of setting powder using this process, as the powder is more likely to fall. Applying is easy, just pat the powder puff over the entire area you have covered with the cream, then leave for about 5 minutes – this is the time I usually dry or style my hair! Once this time has elapsed, use a

HEALTH AND SAFETY ✚

When camouflage make-up is complete, always thoroughly clean the spatula ready for the next use. Inserting a used spatula into the product will transfer bacteria into the product.

brush to clear away any excess or obvious amounts of powder that are superfluous to the make-up, getting into all the nooks, like the sides of the nose, inside the corners of the eyes and the neckline.

9 You are now ready to start your normal make-up routine!

Note from Donna

I complete this make-up regime every day – it takes me approximately three minutes! However, I have been doing it a long time. Take time to apply the make-up in layers, the more slowly and thoroughly you complete a make-up like this, the longer it will last on the model. If you are interested in this type of work, the British Red Cross run courses – or contact me direct, I will be happy to help (see Resources).

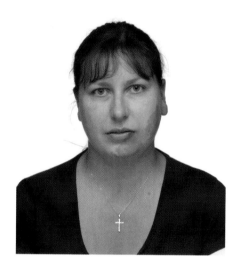

Before from front

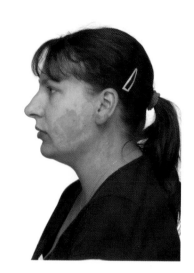

Before from left side

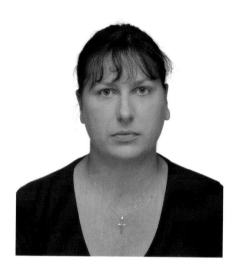

After from front

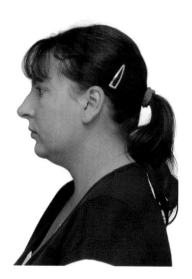

After from left side

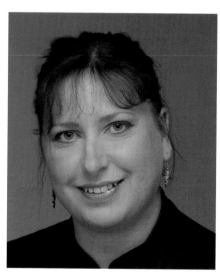

Final look after completion of make-up

Donna's advice for the removal of camouflage make-up from the face: 'It is important to cleanse the make-up off at the end of each day, as the make-up after a while feels like a second skin and can easily be forgotten. They say that it is stubborn and can only be removed with the brand's own cleanser, which isn't strictly true! Over the years I have used everything including soap and water, baby lotion and expensive brands and they all do exactly the same job of getting the make-up off. It is your own preference as to whether they are good enough to remove your particular product and for your particular skin type.'

TATTOO CAMOUFLAGE

Whilst tattoos are fashionable and acceptable in everyday life now, they can become less so on a wedding day or special occasion. Beauty salons are often asked for tattoo camouflage for a big day – both for female and male clients.

1 First check that the skin is clean and clear of any oils or make-up that may affect the application of camouflage creams. Moisturise the skin if it is dry or a dry condition (eczema or psoriasis) is present. Also check for contra indications.

2 Determine the tone (underlying colour) and shade (light or darkness) of the skin or alternatively hold the camouflage palette close to the area to find the closest match. Finding the exact skin tone is the hardest task and you may need to mix several colours together to get it right.

3 Once you think you have the correct match, test it onto the surrounding skin next to the area to be covered. Continue to adjust the skin match if appropriate. When you are happy the skin match is exact, start to apply thin layers of the camouflage directly onto the area, in this case the tattoo. Use a sponge or flat brush and blend the edges just beyond the edge of the area.

4 Apply a fine layer of neutral coloured powder with a sponge or powder puff, and remove excess with a large powder brush.

5 Continue to build the layers with the skin match and powder.

6 As the layers increase, the tattoo will start to disappear. However, occasionally, because tattoos are highly pigmented, they can still be evident under many layers of camouflage. Your next step may be to try colour correction. This involves the use of a colour which is the opposite on the colour wheel to the colour of the area (see Chapter 1): for example, green and red, yellow and purple, blue and orange. Essentially, both colours should counteract each other when used together. Only use the counteracting colour directly on top of the opposing colour displayed, and nowhere else.

7 A tattoo may start to display a slight green tinge at the outline or stronger coloured patterning may still be evident, whilst lighter or softer colours have been disguised. Proceed with the opposing colour, mixed in with the already matched skin tone colour.

8 Continue to use colour correction until the tattoo is covered or finish with a final layer of the skin match and powder to set.

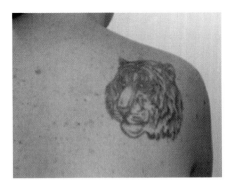

Tattoo removal before

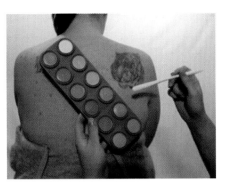

Stage 1 – determine the tone

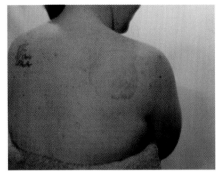

Stage 3 – apply camouflage in layers, setting each layer with neutral powder

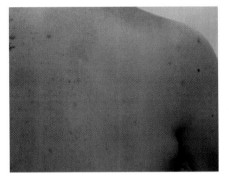

Stages 6 and 7 – use colour correction if required

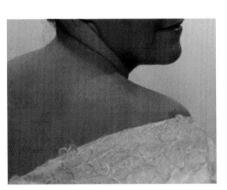

Final overall look

> **TIP** ✔
>
> Be patient in your camouflag work. Several thin layers of make-up may take longer to apply, but the end result will be better, and last longer.

Sometimes it is necessary to use a technique known as 'faking faults'. This is necessary when the camouflaged area looks bland compared to the rest of the natural skin due to the absence of such conditions as freckles, moles, suntan, veins, capillaries, mottled redness, etc. Simply copy the exact colour of the freckles, moles, etc. by random application over the camouflaged area using a brush or stipple sponge. Continue to create these 'faults' until a realistic effect is achieved.

Aftercare

> **TIP** ✔
>
> Always make a note of the colours and quantities of camouflage creams used in case the model wishes to apply the make-up at home.

- Removal of the camouflage cream requires fragrance free creamy cleansers; ones for sensitive skin are useful for some conditions and damp cotton wool is good for wiping off the cream. A mild toner, such as rosewater with a little witch hazel or glycerine, can follow this. Cotton buds can also be used for small areas and disposed of.

- Activities such as sunbathing, swimming and sweat will reduce the durability of the application.

- Ensure clothes are loose and do not rub the area.

- Camouflage products are usually waterproof or water-resistant. After bathing, ask the model to pat the area dry, do not use cosmetics on the area and re-apply powder to reset.

COMMON SKIN CONDITIONS REQUIRING CAMOUFLAGE

Vitiligo

Vitiligo is a pigmentation disorder in which melanocytes in the skin, the mucous membranes and the retina are destroyed. As a result, white patches of skin appear on different parts of the body, known as areas of de-pigmentation. The hair that grows in areas affected by vitiligo usually also turns white. The cause of vitiligo is not known, but doctors and researchers have several theories. One theory is that people develop antibodies that destroy their own melanocytes. Another theory is that melanocytes destroy themselves. Finally, some people have reported that a single event such as sunburn or emotional distress triggered vitiligo; however, these events have not been scientifically proven.

People who have vitiligo, particularly those with fair skin, should use a sunscreen that provides protection from both the UVA and UVB forms of ultraviolet light. Sunscreen helps to protect the skin from sunburn and long-term damage. Sunscreen also minimises tanning, which makes the contrast between normal and de-pigmented skin more noticeable.

Vitiligo can be covered with stains, camouflage make-up or self-tanning lotions, and are particularly effective for people whose vitiligo is on the face and hands.

Chloasma

Chloasma, also known by the name melasma, is a pigmentation disorder usually occurring in patches, anywhere over the body, including the face. Its main cause is hormonal and it occurs most commonly in women, either during pregnancy or through the menopausal years or whilst taking the oral contraceptive pill. The condition is aggravated by sunlight. After a pregnancy, at the end of the menopausal years or when coming off the pill, the pigmentation disorder usually corrects itself. The main characteristic of chloasma is that it shows as brown patches, compared with the white patches of vitiligo.

When choosing a foundation for someone with facial chloasma, do not be tempted to go too dark, to match the dark patch of de-pigmented skin – if anything this will just draw even more attention to the face. Choose one shade darker than you would normally choose, and draw attention to other areas of the face. If, for example, the chloasma patch is over the forehead, choose one shade darker foundation, to blend the patch in a little, and then go for distinctive lips, which will draw attention away from the forehead.

Assessment of knowledge and understanding

Knowledge review

1 How do camouflage products differ from ordinary cosmetics?

2 What pigmentation and skin disorders can be covered by camouflage make-up?

3 What is the most important aspect of camouflage make-up?

4 What is a port wine stain?

5 What is 'faking faults'?

6 What is vitiligo?

7 Can vitiligo be covered with camouflage make-up?

8 What is chloasma?

9 Can chloasma be covered with camouflage make-up?

10 What are the main differences between a fashion make-up artist and a camouflage make-up artist?

chapter 13

Face and body painting

Body and face painting, and cave art, were probably the earliest forms of human artistic expression. It was practised by a diverse range of cultures and on most continents, from the Americas to Australia. We cannot be certain why prehistoric people developed this art, but one reason may have been to mark momentous occasions in life. Body art may have been used to mark a person's death and departure to the afterlife, for example, or to represent beliefs when undertaking a difficult hunt or journey, or to make warriors look fierce in battle. Today, we practise the art of tattooing and body painting for decorating bodies, and fantasy face painting where children and adults can 'realise' their dreams. The dream could be that of a young boy who wishes to show he is a strong powerful masculine creature – he could choose to be a lion, a tiger or a monster. A girl may wish to 'realise' her femininity, choosing a princess, which gives her power and beauty, and allows her to wear make-up just like mum!

Learning objectives

In this chapter you will learn about:

- **health and safety issues connected with body painting**
- **the materials used in body painting to achieve a desired effect**
- **techniques used for face and body painting**
  - **application of paint using sponges**
  - **stippling**
  - **application of paint using brushes**
  - **methods of 'edging' a face**
- **face and body painting designs**
  - **monsters and dragons**
  - **tribal body 'tattoo'**
  - **black and gold design**
  - **fantasy cat**
  - **daisy eye design**
- **body painting designs**
  - **frog prince**
  - **spine and muscles**
  - **necklace**
  - **St George's flag**
  - **Road to Oz**
  - **total body gold**
- **introduction to airbrushing**

HEALTH AND SAFETY

It is important to observe all health and safety regulations when applying any type of body or face painting. Avoid contact with the inside of the eyes, ears and nostrils and be aware of cross contamination of the equipment used.

Face and body painting can take a long time to complete. The artist should be aware of his or her working position and should be comfortable at all times, and the make-up process must be carried out so as to minimise discomfort to the model. If it is a long procedure (a full body paint can take 3–5 hours), check that the working environment is well ventilated, but also warm enough for the model, who may be wearing very little clothing. Do not get so involved with the work that you forget to take frequent small breaks for water and food consumption.

FACE PAINTING

Materials used in face and body painting

Traditionally, paints were made out of berries, bark, leaves and earth, which were ground and then mixed with vegetable oils or animal fat. Today water paint, known as aqua paint, is the most frequently used material for face and body painting. These are water-soluble paints that can be removed easily.

Face painting is a bold art form, where contrast is really important. Face painting must work both close up and from a distance, so it needs to be a compromise between the fineness of fashion and photographic work and the power of theatre, although it should not be crudely executed.

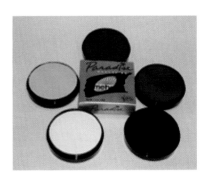

Paradise Aqua colours

Due to the time constraints that working with children entails, face painting can also be a reasonably speedy make-up style. Strong powerful brush strokes are a must and are where the real skill of the face painter comes into play. A quality brush, one that is responsive and holds its point well, is invaluable. Good quality aqua make-up is important too.

Techniques for face and body painting

Application of paint using sponges

When applying face paint with a sponge, it is important to get the consistency of the make-up right. Generally, streaks in the application are from the product and/or the sponge being too wet.

Unlike the latex sponges used in applying traditional foundation products, the sponges used in face painting should be of an open texture making them more porous. This will allow some of the paint to be stored inside the sponge. The shape of the sponge is one of personal choice, with many painters enjoying the circular sponges. However, if you cut the sponge in

TIP
The easiest way to add water is to use a spray/misting bottle to either wet the sponge or the make-up.

half, it gives you greater flexibility and double the number of sponges, making it a very cost-effective exercise! It also gives you curves and straight edges to work with which can be more manageable. The cutting should be in one movement with a good sharp pair of scissors. The most successful method of applying the make-up is in small circles, using only enough pressure to transfer the paint from the sponge to the face; this minimises streaks, as you tend to blend them in as you rub around. It is important when applying make-up to a face to cover the whole face if that is your intention, so attention to detail around the eyes and nose is encouraged, pressing the make-up onto the skin below the eyebrows also helps to cover them. In most designs, eyebrows can spoil the overall effect, so you need the eyebrows to be covered with paint to minimise their impact.

Stippling

Stippling is one term used for applying the face or body paint onto the skin's surface. Stippling is the continuous dabbing of the paint from the sponge to the face/body, which leaves the effect of a mottled/speckled finish to the skin.

Application of paint using brushes

When using this make-up with a brush, the consistency of the paint should be slightly thicker than with a sponge. The paint will have to be 'worked' into a creamy consistency, so you can either do this in advance of a painting or as you go, alternatively you could use a fluid make-up instead. The brush needs to be well loaded, to allow you to create long or many lines with one dip into the pot. As face painters use strong line work, it helps if you balance your brush hand to give greater control, it also helps when the model moves – remember some of your models will be children, who cannot sit still for long. Use your little finger to support your brush hand, this gives you the ability to paint a wide full arc with total control (see cat step by step photos).

Methods of 'edging' a face

'Edging' a face means determining the boundaries of the face painting. There are two methods commonly used – a strong edge or a blended edge. To create a strong edge, simply use the straight edge of a sponge well loaded with make-up and, with a little pressure from your finger, 'draw' a line around the edge of the face – your paint will not go beyond this boundary. When choosing a blended edge, use the method for the strong edge to do a small part and then blend outwards towards the hair, gradually working around the face, taking the make-up into the hair and painting right through the hair – effectively bringing the hair into the painting.

You can bring any colours into your painting that you feel are right, in order to create the effect you want.

How and when did you start in the business?

After 20 years as a calligrapher and heraldic artist, I decided to retrain as a make-up artist. I completed NVQ Level 2 hairdressing and wig making but I felt that it wasn't an appropriate field of work for me. A professional magician I was working on in the theatre said 'You can earn a living as a face painter' – well that was 3¹/₂ years ago. I am happy with my choice as it fits in with my family commitments.

Was there a turning point in your career?

Seeing the first edition of *The Face Painting International* magazine, seeing Oliver Zeger's work and bringing him over to the UK to teach. I met many new friends, with him amongst them, as well as learning to paint each face with thought and consideration for the shape and contours of the face and using colour to an advantage.

What do you consider to be important qualities for a professional face painter?

Personality, good manners, an enjoyment of people and an ability to communicate are important qualities for a professional painter. The same qualities are needed for make-up artists generally.

What is your most memorable/exciting/best paid job?

Best paid – a one-hour film premier! Most memorable and exciting – working on a tour with two great friends.

Have you had any disasters?

Not in jobs as such – the odd face – yes!

What advice would you give to anyone entering the industry?

It may seem glamorous but it's still long hours and hard work – albeit rewarding.

In your experience, would you advise those training to become make-up artists to specialise in one area only, or to gain experience, through Continued Professional Development courses (CPD) in many different areas of make-up?

Never stop training/learning – it is your best tool. Nothing in this business stands still. It's also a great way to network and make new friends.

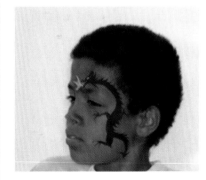

Dragons are also a favourite for boy face painting

Here are some simple face painting examples. Do not copy these paintings exactly, but try to create your own by using different colours, your imagination and the principles being described.

Monsters and Dragons

1 Apply colour with a sponge to half the model's face, adding the paler colour to represent the protruding points of the monster design. Blend these colours together with the sponges if you want a softer edge. Untidy edging at this stage isn't a worry, as it will be outlined.

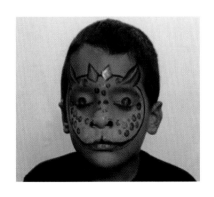

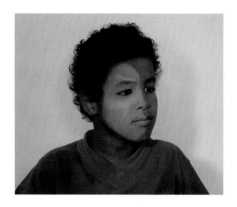

Monster boy 1

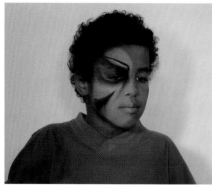

Monster boy 2

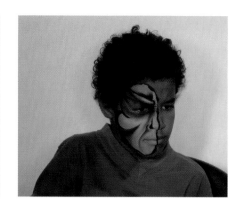

Monster boy 3

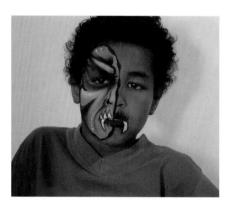

Monster boy 4

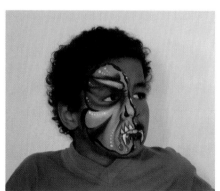

Monster boy 5

2 Create further depth to the face with a dark colour, black in this case, applied with a medium brush. Red has been added with a brush and blended with a sponge to create more warmth and interest.

3 More definition is added with black, again, creating wrinkles and a defined edge. The edge is created using a line of varying thickness. This is done by lifting and then pushing on the medium brush. The variation, again, creates interest. Blending in the smaller areas is done using a dry filbert brush rather than the sponge.

4 Highlights are added with white and blended using a sponge or brush. Further detail/interest is created with dots as texture on the monster's skin. Monster teeth are created using simple brush strokes. The outlining of the upper teeth was created first by blending up with a brush then the white tooth added after. The lower fangs are outlined to define them and to create contrast.

5 Red 'blood' has been added to create a more gory effect; this is still just red make-up rather than stage blood. Where this goes is a matter of choice – the example suggests the monster has just feasted and also as if the 'monster' half of the face is breaking out of the 'human' one. The drops are highlighted with a little white to create the impression of the blood being wet and 3D.

13.1 Start watching any science fiction TV or film and make notes on the variety of face painting designs.

Face painting just for children?

Face painting is often thought of as only enjoyed by the very young, but face and body decoration can be used to great effect on all ages. Study any futuristic or sci-fi series on television and you will see many examples of face painting on adults.

Tribal body tattoo

The blue design on the side of the face and on the front of the body, in our example, is tribal and simple. Clean brush work is the key here, flattering the face and torso, and gold details have been added to create a more luscious look.

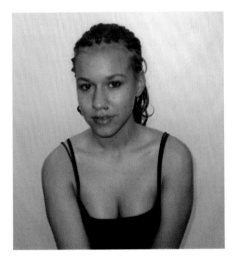

Blue face and body tribal 'tattoo' before

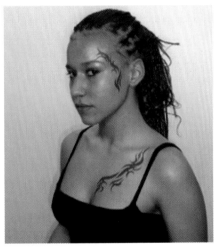

Stage 1 – paint design with blue and gold

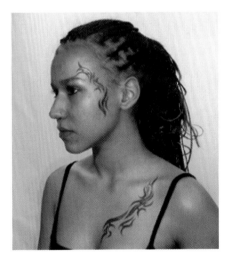

Stage 2 – add gold detail for final look

Black and gold design

The black design shown here on the sides of the face is more feminine and soft. The base is gold aqua paint. Again, strong simple brush strokes, creating teardrops, have been added and then fine lines to link and flow. Some small gold details have also been applied to add interest as the face moves. The lines are placed to flatter the face, the asymmetry is to create a degree of tension and interest. Glitter can be used on both designs, but if applied carelessly could cover them detrimentally.

TIP

An interesting way of getting the sparkle without hiding the line work is to apply the glitter to the base and paint over the top.

TIP

Glitter should be applied to models with braided hair carefully as it is difficult to remove.

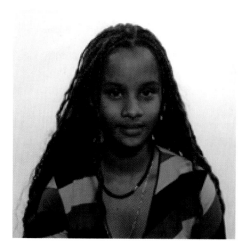

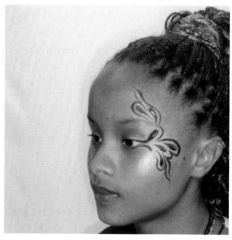

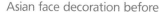

Asian face decoration before

Asian face decoration after

Preparation for painting a Fantasy Cat

Before starting to paint you need to ask yourself 'What are the main characteristics of cats?' Generally speaking these are the muzzle, whiskers, nose and the eyes. The cat's muzzle comes forward and as a prosthetic is not being used, you have to use colour to create the illusion.

1 Using clean sponges for each colour, apply the aqua colour make-up evenly over the face. Start with white on the upper lip to bring it forward, then use two medium tones gradually getting darker as you work towards the outside of the face – thus creating a concave effect. Blue has been used to create interest in the background and to coordinate with the model's shirt. The placement of these colours can be anywhere, but use your knowledge of shaping the face to good effect. Blending the colours together is important if you are going for a soft look, and here the blending has been done with white.

2 The edging of the face has been done with a strong edge, and the lines on the nose are created by drawing the sponge along the edge of the nose. It is necessary to lift the sponge so that only the edge is in contact with the skin. Blending the pink into the face is done by alternating the pink, the yellow and the white sponges.

3 Another important aspect of face painting is the need for contrast – so black is used for the line work. You will need to use a medium round paintbrush and mix the make-up to a creamy consistency. Paint a small neat nose and then the muzzle. To create the illusion of the nose and muzzle coming out of the face, it is important to keep the top lip white; with the black line creating the muzzle edge between the lips and following through in a smooth rounded line. This means the face will still work when the model is talking. Once this line has been painted, the cat's muzzle is created; the white paint giving the impression of the lip coming forward and the black creating a shadow and 'knocking' the lower lip back. The muzzle can be any shape or size, from a small curly one to a large angular one. The important lines are those that create the split lip and the edge of the lips. The black lines can be blended to create a softer look.

4 Prepare the tip of your brush into a fine point, and load with paint to paint in teardrops. Teardrops are created by placing the tip of the brush on the face and as you draw the brush back you increase the pressure on the bristles, pushing the body of the brush down onto the face. The placement of these lines/patterns is at the face painter's discretion but where you place them is important and the face structure must be carefully considered. In this cat face we are looking to flatter, so the lines work with the 'pretty' lines in the face. Different placements would be chosen for a bad tempered grouchy cat.

5 To create further contrast and to lift the face, whiskers, dots and teeth are added in white paint. The dots are created by overloading the top of the brush and literally dotting paint onto the face. For the whiskers, you can either change to a finer brush or, just create a point on the medium round brush and paint a fine line. The teeth are created with one stroke too, pressing the brush onto the lip and pulling it off the face as you draw down. It is important to outline the teeth and lower lip to create a finished look and to underline the whiskers with white to create the impression of them going over the lip.

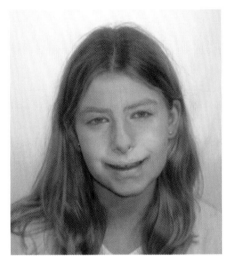
Fantasy Cat 1

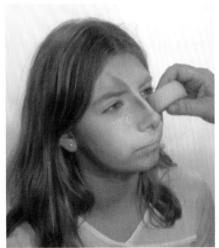
Fantasy Cat 2

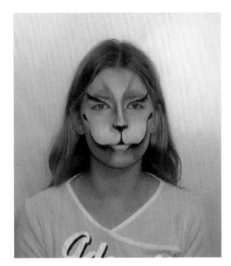
Fantasy Cat 3

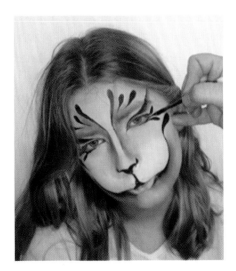
Fantasy Cat 4

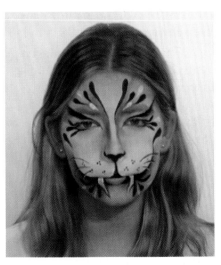
Fantasy Cat final

TIP

Take care when blending colours – if you are blending blue and yellow for example, you do not want to end up with green – so take a little white on a clean sponge and blend the two colours together – this will give a soft look.

6 If glitter is being used, now is a good time to use it. Apply it with caution as it could hide the details and beauty of the face you have painted if it is applied all over.

7 As it is usual practice for models not to watch as the design is being painted, the final step is to show the model their face in the mirror and enjoy the reaction!

STUDENT ACTIVITY

13.2   Start looking at cats' faces, including lions and tigers, and note the various shapes and sizes. If you intend to start painting animal faces, collect pictures and cuttings and file in a logical order.

Daisy eye design

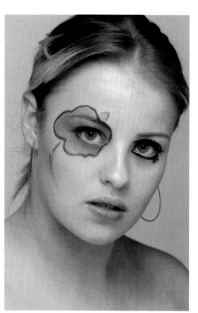

Twiggy 'eye' painting

We now look at a famous 1960s face painting design, originally painted on Twiggy.

This design has an airbrushed foundation with the eye design hand drawn using standard make-up.

How to do this look:

1 Conceal if necessary and then airbrush a light base of pale silicon based foundation to the entire face, extending the spray area to the shoulders and **décolletage**. Set with translucent powder. Airbrush a light pink blush to the cheeks.

2 Cover the entire left eye lid up to the eyebrow with a white matt powder eye colour and define the left eyebrow with light brown powder and set with clear gel.

3 Draw a flower shape over the right eye using a red liner or red cream eye shadow and a small brush. Ensure the entire right eyebrow is encapsulated. Fill in the shape with an even coat of light blue cream dye shadow. Draw in a leaf and flower stem detail using pale green liner or cream shadow with a small brush. Accentuate the shading and detail with darker green.

4 Apply spike thick false eyelashes to both eyes and line the upper lash line of both eyes with black liquid liner. Using black liquid liner, draw an exaggerated crease on the left eye above the actual crease line and extend down to the outer edge of the eye. Encircle the bottom lash line and draw the false eyelashes on the outer edge of the eye. Apply black mascara to the upper lashes of both eyes.

5 Line the lips with pale pink lip pencil and fill in.

6 Finish with clear lip gloss.

You could use the same principles for painting a witch as you would when applying make-up for ageing for instance. Caricature the designs and pick the main characteristics that make that face. Vary the colours you use and match the face to the model's clothing. The only limit to the faces you paint will be your imagination.

MAKE-UP ARTIST PROFILE: ANN EATWELL

How and when did you start in the business?

In 1999 I studied and gained a diploma in Theatrical and Media Studies. In that same year I was invited to body paint in the European Body Painting Festival that is held annually in Seeboden in Austria, and then there was no turning back.

Was there a turning point in your career?

The Festival combined with being invited to teach Theatrical and Media Make-Up at South Kent College. I had taken my teaching certificate in 1997 and gained an Honours degree in Education in 2000.

What do you consider to be important qualities for a professional face painter?

A make-up artist must be patient and not mind working irregular hours. They should also be able to put models at their ease. An artist also needs to be confident in their skills, have a creative flair and an eye for detail.

What is your most memorable/exciting/best paid job?

I was asked to paint Nell McAndrew for a promotion for the British Heart Foundation. I gave my services for free, partly because I believed that this was an opportunity to not only upgrade the 'Body Painting' image, but also give me great advertising, which I could never otherwise have afforded. I was asked to submit two prototype designs painted on my own models and they chose the second one. The 'shoot' was held in October 2003 in London ready for the promotion in February 2004. As the body paint would have taken 3–4 hours I was asked if I had a colleague who would help with the painting. I asked my friend Jackie Brisley whom I have often worked with and we shared the painting and managed to complete it in less than 2 hours. It was a day neither of us will ever forget. The photographer was Jeannie Savage and the photos were brilliant. The only trouble was that although we were given the practice, we were not allowed to take any photos and could not be given any until after the promotion. It was a national promotion so featured in every British Heart Foundation charity shop and a picture of Nell was in the *Daily Record* on 16th February 2004. Photos can be seen on my web site (see resources).

What advice would you give to anyone entering the industry?

To network, give your time for free initially to gain lots of experience – such as school plays, local theatres, face painting at fetes – and then just enjoy!!!

In your experience, would you advise those training to become make-up artists to specialise in one area only, or to gain experience, through Continued Professional Development courses (CPD) in many different areas of make-up?

Although most of my students seem to want to specialise in one area, I always advise that they gain experience in a variety of different areas to build up their skills.

BODY PAINTING

The models' comfort is always paramount as a body paint will, normally, take between 3 and 5 hours. After ensuring that your model is not sensitive to the paint, make sure she or he is moisturised all over. To assist the comfort of your model, lay down something warm and soft to stand on and make certain the environment is warm enough for her or him to be naked. Also make sure that water is available at all times for your model to drink. It is not easy standing still for that length of time.

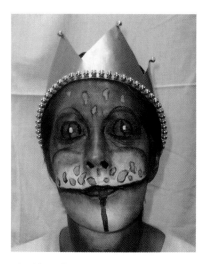

Final head – Frog Prince

EQUIPMENT AND PRODUCT LIST

Equipment and products for the Frog Prince

Equipment

Body painting brushes: large, medium, small, fine brush

Blending brush

Round painting sponge

Stamper (e.g. a rose)

Products

Paradise body paints

Black, dark green, red, violet, white, purple

Mehron fixing liquid

Mehron gold metallic powder

Snazaroo pearl green

Snazaroo silver glitter gel

TIP

Stampers are rubber stamps usually used for making designs on cards, or stamping envelopes and can be bought from most good stationery shops.

Full body painting of Frog Prince

1 Outline the design on the model using a medium brush with white paint (often, with another colour painted on top, this outline can give an added natural highlight).

2 Using a round painting sponge and violet paint, fill in the outline of the jacket using a stippling (dabbing on the paint with the paint filled sponge) motion. Mix up a quantity of the gold metallic powder with the fixing liquid, and apply with the large body painting brush into the outline of the breeches. Using this same gold paint and with a small brush, fill in the outline of the buttons on the jacket on the front, back and the sleeves. With the large brush and pearl green paint, apply to the legs and feet below the breeches and also to the hands. With the medium brush and white paint fill in the ruffle of the shirt and the sleeve cuffs.

3 Using the round painting sponge and purple paint, give another coat to the jacket using a stippling motion. Using the small brush, mix a little black paint with a little of the white paint to create grey. Paint shadows in the ruffles of the shirt-front and the shirt cuffs. Use fingers or a blending brush to blend this in. Using a little black paint, mix with a little of the purple paint and with the small brush create folds under the arms, across the sleeves and on the back of the jacket where they would be relevant. Use your (clean) fingers or a blending brush to blend where appropriate. Also edge the jacket with this mixture of paint. Mix a little of the gold metallic paint with a little of the black paint and do relevant creases in the bottom of the breeches, up the side seams and other relevant places. With a medium brush and silver glitter gel, brush in the cummerbund and then add a little black to a little silver glitter gel and make the relevant creases in the belt. With the medium brush and black paint, elongate the gaps between the toes and the fingers blending in the edges.

4 With a fine brush and the black paint, outline the gold buttons, parts of the jacket which would be appropriate to being in dark shadow, the bottom of the breeches and around the neck edge of the shirt. While edging, use a blending brush to blend all the edges to create a 3D effect.

5 Mixing a little white with each of the main colours in turn, create highlights to correspond appropriately to the low lights already painted. Using silver glitter gel, paint with an appropriate stamper, stamp evenly across the jacket to create a textured look – as in brocade material. Using a stamper in this way will give 'depth' to the paint – giving the appearance of material.

6 With the fine brush and black paint, create some creases in the ruffles on the front of the shirt and cuffs, blending in the edges with a blending brush or fingers. Using white paint and a small brush, highlight the gold buttons and the appropriate edge of the jacket where the light will fall when taking a photograph (or from where the light will be coming). Carefully, with a stipple sponge and with a very small amount of the white paint, dab the shoulders and the top of the chest of the jacket to create sheen. This is often not seen in its right context except from a distance. Using a round painting sponge, stipple the face with the pearl green paint.

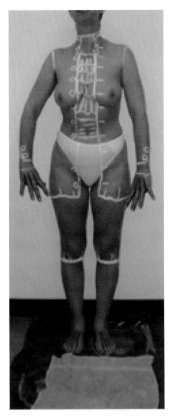

Stage 1 front – Frog Prince

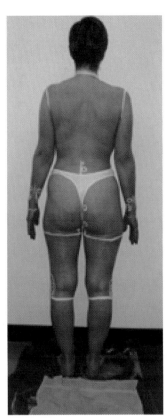

Stage 1 back – Frog Price

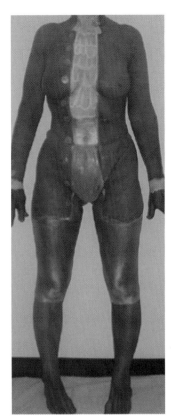

Stage 2 – Frog Prince

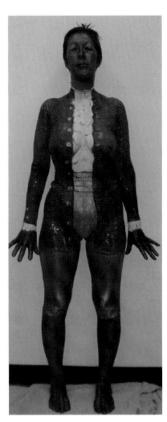

Stage 3 front – Frog Prince

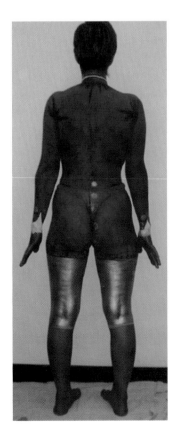

Stage 3 back – Frog Prince

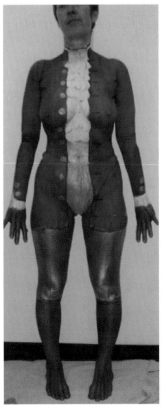

Stage 4 front – Frog Prince

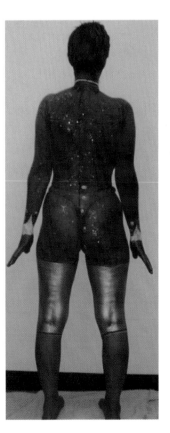

Stage 4 back – Frog Prince

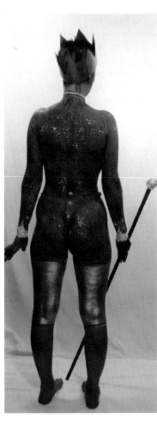

Final back – Frog Prince

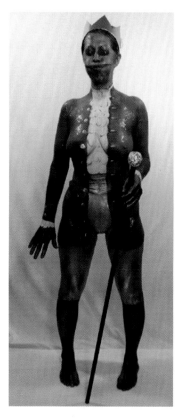

Final front – Frog Prince

EQUIPMENT AND PRODUCT LIST
Equipment and products to paint the Spine and Muscles
Equipment
Body painting brushes: medium, small and fine
Products
Paradise body paints: white, black, red, pink

7 Finish painting the face using red paint for the eyes, mouth and tongue, blending where appropriate. Outline with black and use white for the highlights in the eyes painted on the lids. With a sponge, stipple the top of the face with dark green paint and gold highlights over the chin and muzzle.

8 Always photograph your work upon completion. This can be used as evidence of course work and can also be included in your portfolio.

Part body painting – 'Spine and Muscles'

As an artist, you will have artistic licence for the painting you create, however, for something as explicit as 'Spine and Muscles', it is always advisable to research to make sure that what you design is basically correct. For such exact work, it is imperative that your model can stay very still for minutes at a time, so make sure that the model is comfortable. This body paint can take between $1^{1}/_{2}$ hours and 2 hours to complete.

1 Outline the design on the model, using the medium brush with the white paint.

2 Using the medium brush and the white paint, colour in the bones of the spine and the shoulder blade. Take the small brush and mix a little black paint with the red paint to create a maroon colour for the muscles and colour these in. With the small brush and using the pink paint, fill in between the ribs.

3 Using the small brush, mix a little black paint with a little of the white paint to create grey and blend this in on the appropriate edge of the bones. Now mix a little of the white paint with a little yellow paint and shade the appropriate edges of the bones to give texture and shape. Blend the edges. Take the small brush and mix a little black paint with the red paint to make a darker colour than the maroon of the muscles and shade the appropriate edges, blending the colours in. With the small brush, mix a little of the black paint with the pink paint and shade and blend the pink appropriately between the ribs to give depth.

4 With the fine brush and black paint, outline the appropriate edges of the bones and muscles to give a more 3D effect.

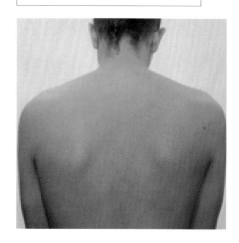

Spine and Muscles before

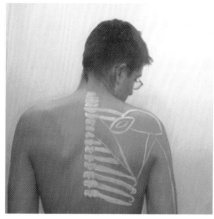

Spine and Muscles stage 1

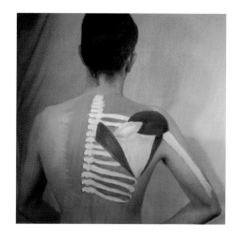

Spine and Muscles final

Necklace body paint

1 Blend the pink with a little water to make a diluted paint mixture. Then, using something such as the cap of a pen or a similar tube dipped into the paint, make circular impressions of the outline of the design around the model's neck.

2 With the small brush and the sparkle white paint, fill in the outline using a circular movement as much as possible.

3 Using the small brush, and again using circular movements, paint pink over the sparkle white, blending in the outline and graduating to the centre of each bead.

4 Using the sparkle white paint and just a minute touch of the pink, blend a mixture with a little water and, with the end of the brush, dot each bead at a position where the light would hit the beads.

5 With the fine brush, blend the pink of the beads into the sparkle white/pink paint of the highlights, leaving a highlight point.

6 This next step is individual, as a colour has to be found or mixed just a shade darker than the model's skin. In this instance, pale brown was blended with just a touch of black. With a fine brush, paint a shadow line under the part of the beads that would be in the dark.

<table>
<tr><td colspan="2">EQUIPMENT AND PRODUCT LIST</td></tr>
<tr><td colspan="2">Equipment and products to paint the Pink Necklace</td></tr>
<tr><td colspan="2">Equipment</td></tr>
<tr><td colspan="2">Body painting brushes – small and fine</td></tr>
<tr><td colspan="2">Products</td></tr>
<tr><td colspan="2">Paradise body paints: pink, white, pale brown, black</td></tr>
<tr><td colspan="2">Snazaroo sparkle white</td></tr>
</table>

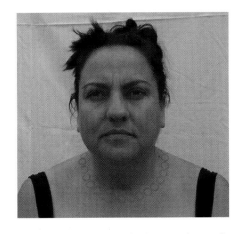

Stage 1 – make circular impressions of the outline of the design around the model's neck

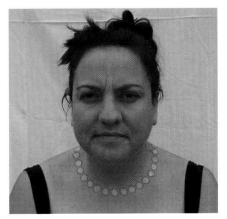

Stage 2 – fill in the outline with white sparkle paint

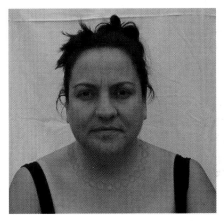

Stage 3 – paint pink over sparkle white

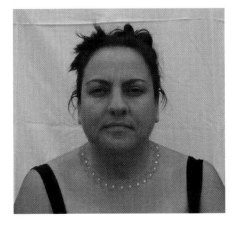

Stage 4 – dot each bead where the light would hit

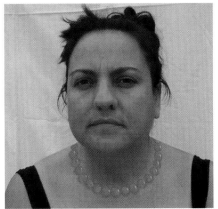

Stage 5 and 6 – blend the highlighted spots and create shadow lines

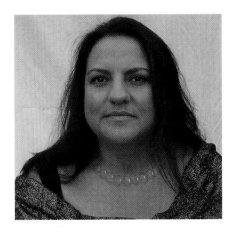

Necklace final

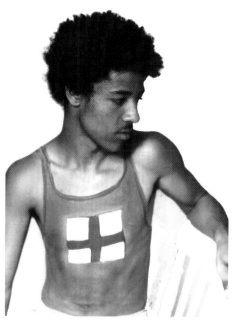

St. George's flag

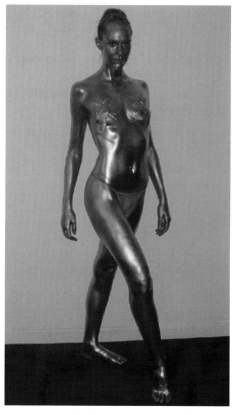

Total body gold

> **TIP**
>
> When body painting try and keep in mind what is beneath what you are painting. For example you can almost 'see' the model's six pack in the St George's flag body painting.

> **TIP**
>
> Don't forget the model when body painting. This total body painting would have taken a couple of hours. Make sure the model doesn't get cold and offer frequent rests.

MAKE-UP ARTIST PROFILE: ALISON WOLSTENHOLME

Make-Up Artist, College Lecturer, Managing Director of Temptu UK – Airbrushing

Was there a turning point in your career?

When I was 18 I took my first professional course in make-up artistry. Back then no make-up was considered complete unless at least fifteen different products had been used on a face, even for day wear. Fashions have changed a lot since then.

What do you consider to be important qualities for a make-up artist?

Apart from creative flair, it would have to be empathy and discretion.

What is your most memorable/exciting/best paid job?

All jobs are exciting because every face is different and every request is different, but mostly I love the buzz of the fashion week catwalk shows.

MAKE-UP ARTIST PROFILE: ALISON WOLSTENHOLME

What advice would you give to young people entering the industry?

Never give up and remember that make-up is temporary so don't panic. If you mess it up, you can always do it again.

In your experience, would you advise those training to become make-up artists to specialise in one area only, or to gain experience, through Continued Professional Development courses (CPD) in many different areas of make-up?

In some geographic areas, companies simply can't afford to employ different make-up artists for every discipline which can make a multi-talented artist a more viable prospect. Having said that, if you find one area you love then stick to it and be the best you can be.

INTRODUCTION TO AIRBRUSHING

Airbrushed make-up has been around for years in the TV and film industries. It was, in fact, first used in the 1922 epic movie 'Ben Hur' where the make-up artists needed to apply make-up to a huge cast. The techniques, equipment and medium have come a long way since then. Everything a make-up artist ever learned about contouring, shading and highlighting still applies, but instead of using sponges and brushes, millions of tiny dots are sprayed onto the face using an airbrush. This lets the natural beauty of the skin shine through. For heavily scarred and imperfect skin, the make-up artist can add extra base to a specific area, no matter how small.

Airbrushing is also useful for prosthetic coverage and the spray will adhere in even coats to any tiny crevasses and hard to reach areas.

The benefits of airbrushing:

- airbrushing leaves the skin with a flawless finish
- it can last 12–24 hours
- it is lightweight
- it is undetectable even under close scrutiny.

Although the application steps are similar to traditional make-up, it is faster and more sanitary because the operator never actually touches the skin. Fantasy and special effects are created quickly with either a freehand or stencilling technique. Colour matching is done through the airbrush, so a make-up artist can dramatically reduce the number of colours and bottles in their kit.

High Definition Television (HDTV) is set to become a big part of our lives with many companies already broadcasting in HDTV. HDTV provides a much sharper picture than analogue television. Just like a digital camera, more pixels mean sharper pictures. The highest resolution HDTV format has approximately 2 million pixels compared to about half a million pixels in analogue TV. This is great for the viewer, but such acute definition shows up every brush line, sponge mark and imperfection. Many people are suggesting some actors look better on HDTV without make-up! Airbrush make-up is a great solution for the make-up artist working in HDTV. It is a fact that many long established make-up artists have lost out on some important jobs because they do not have airbrush make-up experience.

How to airbrush

You will need the right equipment. This requires a dual action, high precision airbrush and an air source, which needs to be in the form of a compressor with an air pressure regulator. The use of a dual action airbrush allows the artist to control the flow of medium used to create heavier or lighter shades, which is invaluable to shading and blending. Regular make-up is not suitable for the airbrush, as it is too thick and will clog the equipment. If the regular make-up is watered down what you get is watered down coverage. There is specially formulated water based airbrush make-up on the market, which dries instantly and gives a matt finish, and a silicon based formulation that gives you two minutes of 'movement time' after application, making it ideal for the mature skin whilst also leaving the skin with a beautiful dewy look.

There are two types of airbrush, dual action and single action. Within these categories they can be gravity or bottle feed. For airbrush make-up on the face, it is recommended to use a dual action gravity feed airbrush, capable of working at low pressure with a 0.3–0.5 nozzle (the thicker the medium the larger the nozzles needs to be). Single action airbrushes don't allow the artist enough control over the flow of medium.

To operate the airbrush you need an air source in the form of a compressor. The compressor should be adjustable and for extended usage have an automatic switch and moisture filter.

Always airbrush in a well-ventilated area. For light to medium airbrushing, that is for one or two people, airbrush by an open window. For more serious body coverage or if there are several artists working at the same time, use a filtered extractor fan to prevent a vapour cloud formation as this can irritate the mucous membranes of the model and artists.

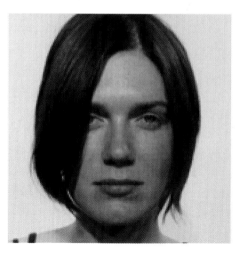

Airbrush foundation and make-up before

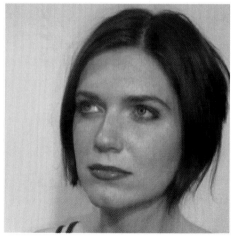

Airbrush foundation and make-up after

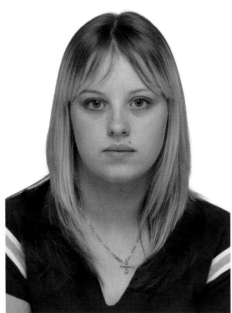

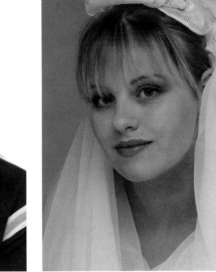

Airbrush bride before   Airbrush bride after

Airbrush bride

1 Conceal any blemished areas and, matching the skin tone, airbrush
  creamy silicon based foundation to the entire face and extend to any
  exposed areas such as décolletage. Check the coverage in natural and
  indoor lighting. Set with powder for a matt effect or leave it as it is for a
  dewy look.

2 Airbrush matt peach water based blush to the cheek apples and highlight
  the temples and cheekbones with a creamy silicon based lighter shade.
  Check the colours in natural and artificial light.

3 Define the eyebrows using a light eyebrow powder and set with clear gel.
  Apply a light dusting of translucent powder to the entire eye lid and then
  airbrush a light base of pale peach eye colour to the entire lid and up to
  the eyebrow line. Airbrush mid-brown or mocha eye colour to the eye
  crease and along the bottom of the eye lid, using a lighter spray to blend
  in. Highlight with palest peach underneath the eyebrow.

4 Define the eyes with mid-brown along the upper lash line and lightly
  along the bottom, soften well. Check the effect in natural and artificial
  light. Apply brown mascara to both upper and lower lashes.

5 Outline the lips with nude pencil and fill in. Apply a peach lip colour over
  the top, blot and re-apply. Everyone wants to kiss the bride, so use several
  light coats for durability and to prevent smudging.

An airbrush tattoo

1 Select the design you want and clean the area of skin where you intend to apply the design with Isopropyl rubbing alcohol (70%) or MediSwabs.

2 Place the tattoo on the slightly damp skin (from alcohol) ink side down and dab the back of the paper with a MediSwab until the design shows through.

3 Pat and press the back of the design to 'transfer' the design from the paper to the skin. Alternate and repeat steps 2 and 3 several times.

4 Lift paper (while still wet) away from the skin to reveal a black ink tattoo.

5 If you want to colour in your design, paint those areas with body paint. Start by edging the design and filling in large areas of block colours. Add shading and highlighting, blending the colours in to each other to complete the look.

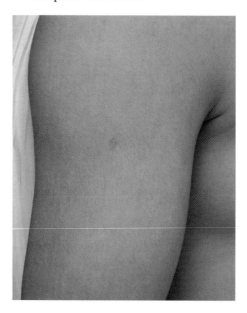

Eagle temporary tattoo before

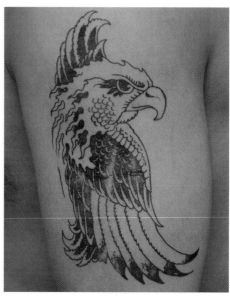

Eagle temporary tattoo stage 1 – the outline is first sprayed onto the cleansed area

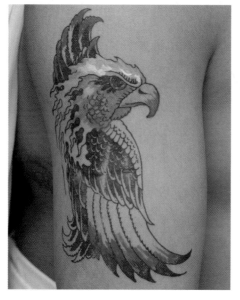

Eagle temporary tattoo stage 2 – first colours are applied

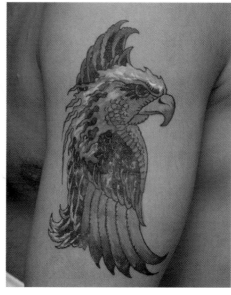

The final look is achieved after adding in the finer details of colour

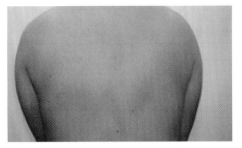

Airbrush back tattoo before

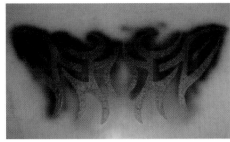

Airbrush back tattoo stencil

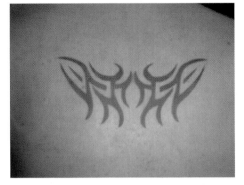

Airbrush back tattoo stage 1

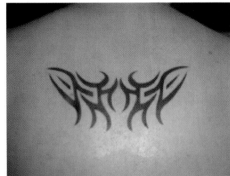

Airbrush back tattoo final

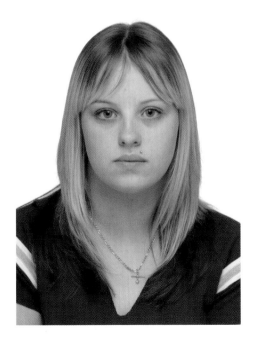

Airbrush mask before

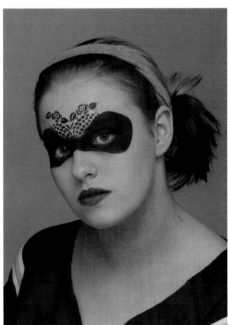

Airbrush mask final

Assessment of knowledge and understanding

Knowledge review

1 What preparations would you make prior to painting a body?

2 Which type of make-up is specifically used for body painting?

3 Which types of tools are used in body painting?

4 When airbrushing, what is the potential health hazard?

5 Describe the type of sponge you would use to create the effect of stippling.

6 Which types of airbrush are available?

7 When is it appropriate to use airbrushing techniques?

8 What would you make in order to create a repeat pattern?

9 Name two benefits of airbrushing.

10 How would you stop a vapour cloud formation when airbrushing?

chapter 14

Mendhi or henna skin decoration

Mendhi is the art of body decorating using henna, a natural colour obtained from leaves. The purpose of traditional henna decorating varies from culture to culture. Henna is most commonly and traditionally used for weddings and bridal preparations, when designs tend to be large and ornate. It is also used for the celebration of circumcision, pregnancy, birth, and for general good luck, friendship and beauty. Sometimes described as temporary tattoos, henna skin decoration is becoming fashionable as a means of self-expression, where designs can be a mixture of traditional and modern. You will need a lot of patience to become a good henna artist and many hours of practice – but the beautiful end results are worth it.

Learning objectives

In this chapter you will learn about:

- **what Mendhi is**
- **assessing a model for Mendhi treatment**
- **preparation of the model**
- **equipment and materials**
- **Arabic, Indian, Sudanese and self-expression design**
- **removal of Mendhi and home care instructions**

WHAT IS MENDHI?

The Indian word Mendhi translates to 'henna' and refers to the art of applying this natural colour onto the skin in intricate designs and patterns. Mendhi has been used since ancient times, but its exact origins are difficult to find. Centuries of migration and cultural interaction make the task of determining henna's exact origin a complex one too. However, historians agree that henna has been used for at least 5000 years in both cosmetic and healing capacities. Some researchers state that henna originated in ancient India, while others claim it was brought to India by the Egyptians. Still others will contend that the tradition of applying henna to the body began in the Middle East and North Africa. We do know, however, that the art of henna decorating has been practised in northern Africa, the Middle East, southern Asia and Europe and has been used by Hindus, Sikhs, Jews, Muslims, Christians, pagans and others.

Mendhi is a henna leaf paste that is applied to the surface of the skin. Henna paste is a semi-permanent dye, which stains only the outer layer of the skin. When applied, the wet henna paste is initially very dark or even black, but the resulting pattern varies from light orange to dark brown. The resulting depth of pattern will depend upon many factors:

- the recipe used
- how long the henna was left on the skin
- the warmth of the room in which the henna was applied.

Once removed, a vibrant, dark orange-brown colour remains on the skin for several days to several weeks, depending on the mixture, the application and how the decoration is looked after. It is not a tattoo, as the practice does not require any piercing of the skin – but the designs are often referred to as temporary tattoos.

ASSESSING A MODEL FOR MENDHI TREATMENT

As with all make-up application, a Mendhi skin decoration needs planning.

- A full consultation must be taken to identify the model's requirements and expectations and to determine the extent to which these can be achieved.
- If there is any history of allergy or intolerance to henna or *any* cosmetic substances, a patch/skin test must be undertaken 24 hours before the service.
- It should be decided at the consultation stage what type of henna you will be using on the treatment day. This will be either a ready mixed preparation of henna or a mix of your own.
- The skin type should be noted from the area to be decorated, and the model should be requested to exfoliate that area before treatment, to ensure a longer lasting design that will be deeper and more even in colour. This is of particular importance for models with dry skin.
- The model should be shown a portfolio of designs at the consultation stage. Once an appropriate design has been chosen, a worksheet will be prepared with the approved design, with any modifications as agreed if applicable. The design may need to be made larger or smaller to take account of body shape and/or size of the model.

HEALTH AND SAFETY

Never apply henna if there has been any adverse reaction to a patch/skin test, or where there are skin disorders.

HEALTH AND SAFETY

Whichever product is chosen for the treatment will be the product with which you do the patch test.

14.1 Design a worksheet

Design a worksheet suitable for a Mendhi decoration service. This should include all the model's details plus the actual design you and the model have decided would be the most appropriate. You may need a separate piece of paper if the design needs to be modified in any way – made larger or smaller than the original design. It is important that the actual size of the design is shown to the model on paper, before commencing on the skin.

Contra indications to a henna skin decoration treatment would include:

- adverse reaction to a patch test
- skin disorders
- cuts or abrasions.

MAKE-UP ARTIST PROFILE: SHABANA BEGUM

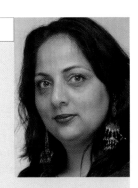

How and when did you start in the business?

Since the age of 16, I worked in factories for several years whilst attending evening classes at college to gain my qualifications in hairdressing and beauty therapy. I started working firstly part time in 1995 and in 2003 started working full time as a freelance artist/therapist. I opened my own business, Aroosa Beauty, in Huddersfield in 2005.

Was there a turning point in your career?

Yes, when I became trainer and distributor with IMPE2US for TEMPTU body art, and being introduced to other very talented make-up artists in the industry.

What do you consider to be important qualities for a make-up artist?

Natural flair and passion for their work. Ability to learn and understand their client's requirements and to be able to learn new and different techniques.

What is your most memorable/exciting/best paid job?

Most memorable was at the age of 13 being asked to do my first ever bridal makeover!

Most exciting and best paid job was when I was hired as a wedding planner to cover a double wedding, not only was that opportunity exciting and challenging, but also it was extremely well paid! Everything was to be perfect for the big day – and it was!

Have you had any disasters?

None so far!

What advice would you give to young people entering the industry?

Look out for opportunities as they will not come your way very often. Keep an open mind and learn as much as possible. Get in touch with a qualified, established artist and see if you can work with them – maybe in an apprenticeship manner. Try to get as much hands on experience as possible, and network – that is the key to success.

In your experience, would you advise those training to become make-up artists to specialise in one area only, or to gain experience, through Continued Professional Development courses (CPD) in many different areas of make-up?

It is ideal to train in your specialised field i.e. as a make-up artist first but then also gain experience in other fields such as stage and television make-up, hairdressing and beauty therapy as they all complement each other. The more knowledge you gain the more versatile and aware you are of the latest trends. The best way of gaining experience and knowledge is to continue with learning. There is always something new to learn.

PREPARATION OF THE MODEL

Leave enough time to prepare the model and yourself fully, before commencing the treatment. Henna decoration cannot be rushed.

- Exfoliation is strongly recommended and may be offered as an additional part of the treatment – the day before decoration if possible.
- Suitable cleansing for different skin types is important, as this can prolong the life of the design. Use a non-alcoholic cleansing agent.
- Provide the model with a protective covering for areas not being decorated.
- Jewellery should be removed from areas to be decorated.
- Everything you need for the decoration should be to hand. The materials to be used should be stored at the correct temperature and have been freshly and hygienically prepared.
- The model's chosen and approved design should be to hand – signed by the model confirming the size and design of decoration.

EQUIPMENT AND MATERIALS

Henna cones

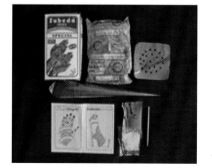

Mendhi products

Although there are different ways to apply henna, plastic homemade cones make good applicators. You can buy ready made application bags with plastic tips but these can become expensive. Try different cones until you

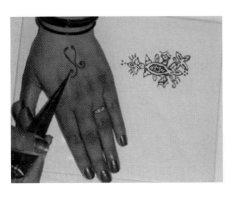

Sequence 1 – always have the original design to hand before you start

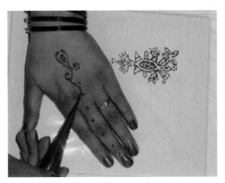

Sequence 2 – apply marker points to work

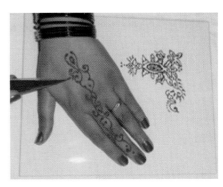

Sequence 3 – using your marker points, fill in decoration

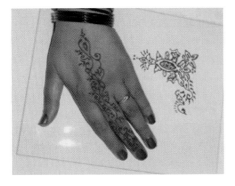

Sequence 4 – complete one area at a time

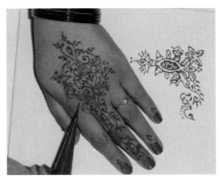

Sequence 5 – nearing completion

find one you work well with. In the meantime, try making some out of plastic freezer bags. Do not cut the bottom tip until you are ready to start applying the henna.

1 Cut 18–22cm squares out of plastic freezer bags.

2 Roll corner inside to create cone shape.

3 Wrap corner around cone.

4 Adjust cone until the point is closed, tape flat.

When rolling a cone, it needs to be closed as tight as possible at the tip. You can then determine your application point once it is filled with henna. Simply trim the long tip off with scissors. Progressively trim more if necessary, depending upon the width or size of the line or design you want. Creating several cones for one application will save you valuable time.

Cone fillers

These are usually zip locked bags of ready prepared henna. Make a 1cm cut in the corner of the henna filled bag and fill the ready made application cone, or your homemade cone to approximately half full. Avoid over filling. Fold over each side of the cone, and then over the middle. Be sure to fold the plastic tightly against the henna in the tube. Tape down and seal top.

EQUIPMENT AND PRODUCT LIST
Equipment and materials for making plastic henna cones
Heavy plastic sheeting (such as freezer bags)
5 cm plastic packaging tape or masking tape
Scissors

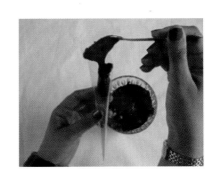

Filling the henna cone

TIP

Be sure you are using mendhi henna, not hair henna for best results.

HEALTH AND SAFETY ✚

Under no circumstances use black henna if it contains paraphenylene diamine (PPD), and this can cause server dermatological problems.

TIP

If you keep the mixing utensil in the mixture, you will not create bubbles. Only when you repeatedly lift the mixing utensil out of the mixture, as when beating eggs for example, will you create bubbles.

TIP

Tamarind, tea, coffee and lemon are known as mordents in henna skin decoration. Mordents are chemical catalysts that help activate the henna.

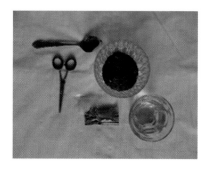

Equipment to make henna

Henna for immediate use

Ready mixed henna is available, but always check the 'best before' dates and correct storage conditions. Old batches can result in a light colour.

Henna powder

The freshest henna is a green powder. Ask for the henna powder to be pre-sifted. You will know if you need to sift the powder if there are small traces of sediment, such as leaf stems, and if it feels grainy between your fingers. Henna is a very sensitive product to work with, and having fine henna powder is essential for a good mix. Coarse henna will not fit through your cone tip. Follow the manufacturer's instructions, if there are any, but always take care to mix with the minimum of air bubbles. The henna leaves need to be treated carefully so that optimum colour will result. This takes time, so patience is needed, as henna has to have time to develop (cure). There are no exact recipes for henna, so trial, error and experience are also needed. Basically you will need to add to the henna powder something to activate the henna and make the colour darker, for example tamarind, coffee or tea, and boiling water. Once applied to the skin, no matter how dark the henna, if the room you are working in is not warm, then a light colour will result. Henna needs, and traditionally has, developed in warm climates: India and Morocco for example. So always apply in a warm environment.

Lemon juice and sugar

If a darker design is required, this can be safely provided by dabbing the completed design with lemon juice and sugar and leaving to dry.

Mordents

Tamarind, coffee or tea may be mixed with the henna paste, before application to produce a safe, but darker effect.

Henna recipes

There are many recipes for henna and it is recommended you experiment with several until you find one you really like to work with. Whichever recipe you choose, the most important ingredient is good quality henna. It should be fresh and green. The brighter the green, the fresher the henna. And, to avoid clogs, your henna should be finely sifted; the powder should be the consistency of talcum powder. A little henna goes a long way; as little as 1 tablespoon of mixed henna will be sufficient for a whole hand decoration. Your proportions should be roughly one part henna powder, 2 parts liquid and $\frac{1}{2}$ part sugar.

Here is a tried and tested henna recipe:

- 1 part henna powder – fresh and green
- 2 parts boiling liquid

- 3 tea bags
- Sugar

Make a mug of regular tea (no milk or sugar) using 2 or 3 tea bags and boiling water. Put the boiling tea into a large bowl and gently stir in the henna powder until a yoghurt like consistency occurs. Adjust with more boiling water or more powder to reach the right consistency. Ladle the henna into a plastic freezer bag – do not pour as air bubbles may be created. Place the henna in a dark place to set. When the top layer turns dark green, the henna is activated and ready for use. This will take a minimum of 2 hours, but peak colour will take from 24 to 48 hours to develop. To get the best from your henna mix, avoid exposure to air and light.

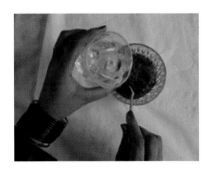
Adding water to henna

HEALTH AND SAFETY ✚

Take care when using boiling water.

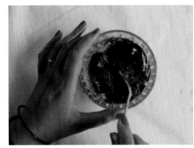
Mixing the paste

DESIGNS FOR HENNA DECORATION

There are four principal design styles in henna painting:

- Arabic designs feature large patterns on the hands and feet.
- Indian designs are more intricate with fine-lines and 'paisley' patterns that have dense design and detail. In a wedding decoration, often the new husband's name is hidden in the design. Hearts and peacocks (which are a sign of luck) are also popular.
- Sudanese designs are large and bold with geometric angles.
- Self-expression designs can be a mixture of all the above and are personalised for individual tastes. Symbols that have a significant meaning to the model are often used: religious or spiritual symbols (crosses, ankhs, Om's, etc.) or script writing from other cultures (Runes, Chinese characters, Arabic, Tibetan or Sanskrit, etc.). Others choose designs purely for aesthetic purposes, like trailing vines or filigree patterns. The potential variety in design is practically limitless.

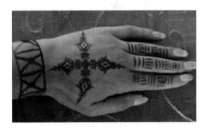
Traditional Sudanese design

Designs and symbols are usually decorated on the hands, feet, arms, legs and torso. There is no particular reason why faces may not be the subject of henna skin decoration, although at this time it is not common.

Feet of the Guru

Hand of Fatima

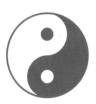
Yin Yang

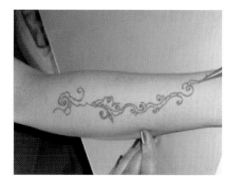

Hand/arm design – starting the design

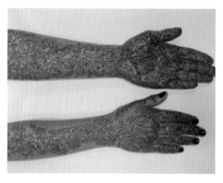

Hand/arm design – completed

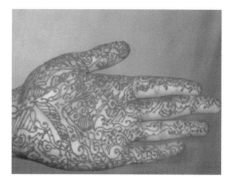

Hand/arm design – close up of hand design

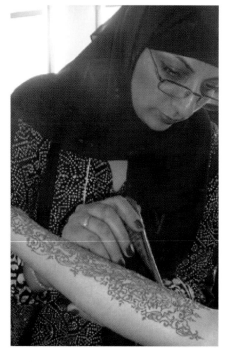

Shabana – working on a leg design

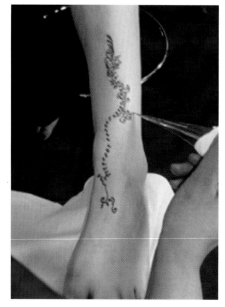

Stage 1 of the leg and foot design

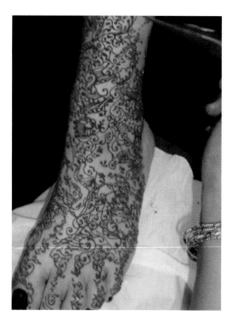

Leg and foot design

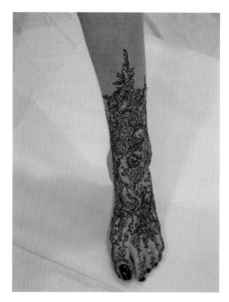

Leg and foot design – completed

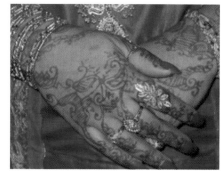

Bridal hand

HOME CARE ADVICE AND REMOVAL OF MENDHI

The following after care advice should be given to all models:

- wear loose clothing to avoid rubbing the design – ideally for up to 48 hours after application
- keep the design dry for 12 hours after application – or as long as you possibly can
- avoid smudging from 30 minutes to 2 hours after application
- 12 hours after application, moisturise design frequently.

The Mendhi design will just wear away naturally. The design may last from a few days to a few weeks, depending on how well it is looked after. Models can be advised to use an exfoliating cream/scrub to remove remnants of the design when it has begun to deteriorate.

Assessment of knowledge and understanding

Knowledge review

1 From what is natural henna obtained?

2 Name three traditional uses of henna.

3 How many layers of the skin does the henna stain?

4 What is the purpose of performing a skin test prior to a henna treatment?

5 What could you recommend the model carry out prior to a henna treatment, to elongate the life of the design?

6 Name two other means of preparing the model for henna treatment on the treatment day.

7 Name two contra indications to a henna skin decoration.

8 What is the usual breakdown of a henna recipe?

9 How would you know if the henna powder had not been sifted?

10 What is a mordent? Give three examples.

11 What is the minimum time henna will take to develop?

12 What after care advice would you give following a henna decoration treatment?

13 How many principal design styles are there in henna painting? Name them all.

14 Peacocks are often found within a henna design – what do peacocks represent in India?

15 Why should you not use black henna?

chapter 15

Career options

During your training in make-up, you will no doubt have looked forward to particular areas of the syllabus more than others, which may give you some indication about the direction you want to take. On the other hand, you may have no idea at all – because you love all aspects of the work! The world of make-up is vast, but there comes a time in our lives when career decisions have to be thought about, and eventually made. This short chapter on career options is here to help you towards some of those decisions, advising you of some of the advantages and disadvantages of each sector of the market.

Learning objectives

In this chapter you will learn about:

- getting a focus
- working in a beauty salon, spa or retail outlet
- working in the world of fashion magazines
  – editorial and advertising
  – fashion shows and music videos
  – catalogues
- working in television, film and theatre
- building a professional portfolio
- test shoots and show reels
- agents
- key skills

GETTING A FOCUS

If you are already studying for make-up qualifications, remember that it is never too early to start thinking about life after you qualify. Ask yourself seriously which areas of make-up work you most enjoy, and whether there are any areas that you really do not like? Do you want to work with make-up on a full-time basis or just part time? The world of make-up and cosmetics is huge and, whilst there are thousands of vacancies in this field, they do not just land on your doorstep – you must apply yourself and find out who is hiring make-up artists and why. Working in the make-up business is very much about **networking**. Research sites on the Internet – there are hundreds of them that all offer something of interest. Two sites of particular importance are www.mandy.com and www.theknowledgeonline.com both of which offer initial free subscription. These sites alert you to the most recent vacant positions in your field. Vacancies for make-up artists are often for short student films. Usually these are for four or five days unpaid work. However, they usually provide food and travel costs *and* are of great importance to you, as you will receive the make-up artists' 'credit' at the end of the film – which of course goes onto your CV. 'Payment' usually also includes a copy of the film on DVD. These are superb opportunities for building up your portfolio and CV. Vacancies from these two websites come through at all times of the day and night and it is not unusual for a make-up artist to be required with only a couple of hours notice! – if you can fill the position and can guarantee to get there on time, the job is most likely yours. Once you get an opportunity like this, it is up to you to prove yourself. Other jobs that are often advertised through mandy.com are for television work. The Knowledge is mostly film work. Fashion jobs are rarely, if ever, advertised through these sites, as fashion work usually goes through agents (see below).

STUDENT ACTIVITY

15.1   Search the Internet for interesting sites on make-up in general and for work opportunities in general.

WORKING IN A BEAUTY SALON, SPA OR RETAIL OUTLET

If you are working towards Level 2 Beauty Therapy and the make-up units were part of the whole qualification, the chances are that you will want to work in a beauty salon or spa. The kind of make-up services offered at these establishments include wedding party make-ups and individual make-up lessons. This is a good choice if you do not want to be involved with make-up all day, as you will also spend much of your time offering other services. The main problem with these areas is that if you love make-up, you will have very little opportunity to expand your skills. If you *really* love make-up, but you don't want to go down the beauty therapy route, consideration should be given to working in a cosmetics retail outlet as a cosmetics sales person. The advantages are that thorough training is often given in-house and you will work with make-up all day. For work in this area, make-up application skills are required, but applicants with good retail selling skills, stock control knowledge and key skills will have an advantage in securing any position.

A big advantage to working in a beauty salon, spa or retail outlet is that you will *not* have to put together a professional portfolio. A disadvantage is that they do not pay well, and you may have to rely on commission from sales to make up your salary.

If you decide you don't want to work in a retail outlet, spa or beauty salon, you need to start putting a professional portfolio together as, without one, finding work in the make-up industry will be all but impossible (see below).

DIFFERENT KINDS OF FASHION WORK

Editorial and advertising

Make-up for fashion looks can either be very dramatic or very natural but, in all cases, the make-up has to be applied *perfectly* – especially for front cover looks.

Fashion shows and music videos

You will be directed when particular themes are required. Sometimes make-up is minimal so that it does not detract from the clothes, at other times the make-up may be 'mad' – depending on the fashion house. Artistic flair will be needed for fashion show work and knowledge of past eras can be invaluable. Often very dramatic make-up is needed for music videos: bold colour, glitter, sequins, and high fashion looks.

Catalogues

Natural looks are usually used for catalogues. Some make-up artists shun this type of work because they cannot demonstrate their artistic flair and the work may become boring as it involves doing one natural make-up after another. However, catalogue houses often choose exotic locations for their photo shoots – which can compensate for the unimaginative make-up skills required. Having said that, foundation application needs to be perfect and that is a skill in its own right. Artistic flair is not really called for in this area. To attract make-up artists into this field, the pay is often very good.

Working in television

Make-up artists working in television generally make-up presenters and guests for general television work, but they also need experience of period looks for historical programmes. Daytime TV shows often have 'make-over' sessions where a member of the public is given a new look or has a specific fashion make-up problem solved by a team of 'experts'. Television make-up artists working for soap operas need to be diligent about keeping continuity records. With many of the soaps having almost daily showings, and with the actors often filming out of sequence, the continuity sheets are of the utmost importance. The most crucial aspect of working in television, however, is to be able to work as part of a team. An advantage of working in television is that you meet talented and interesting people. However, a disadvantage is that you often have to get up at 4.00am to get to the studios in time for a shoot. When working on a TV film there may be no time for a social life!

Working in the film and theatre industry

If your love of make-up extends to Level 3 work, and you enjoy doing character changes, wigs, postiche and prosthetics work, then you may be destined for a career in theatre, film or television. If this is your love then you will need, in the first instance, to join theatrical groups and offer your services free of charge. This allows you to gain valuable experience from others already working in the field. It is an area where, to get paid work, you will have to produce a professional portfolio of your work and a good CV showing what experience you have. Work in this area can be found from www.mandy.com. Jobs as 'runners' or make-up assistants are also often on this site. A runner is basically a junior within the department who runs all over the place taking messages, getting the coffee, cleaning the make-up brushes, and all sorts of 'important' tasks. A job as a runner is an excellent opportunity to meet people and start networking. The key make-up artist in film work is called the make-up designer. This person is responsible for all the research, design and execution of make-up and hair on a major film production. He or she must choose and supervise all members of the make-up and hair departments allocated to the production, making sure that the required style is achieved. You can set your sights on high flying jobs like this, but you must also be realistic and first do your 'training' as a make-up assistant, gradually moving up the hierarchy ladder.

BUILDING A PROFESSIONAL PORTFOLIO

Putting together your professional portfolio, known as your 'Book' in the trade, is of the utmost importance if you want to get, and to stay, in work. Whilst evidence of successful paper qualifications are, of course, important, your 'Book' is just as, if not, more important. The first thing an agent or any prospective employer will ask is to see your Book. If the contents of your Book are good, and in the style they are looking for, *then* they may well ask you what qualifications you have.

Your Book should only represent your very best work. As your work gets better and you get more experienced, you should remove old work from your Book and replace it with new up-to-date material. If you have an agent, then your Book will stay with the agent, who will, in turn, send it to prospective photographers or fashion houses – often by courier to get your Book there before any one else's, and to ensure that it does not get lost or damaged.

Your Book does not need to include every piece of work you have ever done. Twelve to fourteen photographs of your best, most recent and appropriate work will give a good overview of your style. Don't put 'blood and guts' casualty simulation photographs in your portfolio if you want fashion work, and vice versa. Keep the images relevant to the work you want to do. It is recommended that the first images in the Book are strong and bold and the last pictures also strong with the others in the middle.

When you first start out you may, like many others, be in a 'Catch 22' situation. You can't get work because you don't have a good enough Book to show agents or photographers and you can't get a Book together, because you can't get work! The answer for many make-up artists starting out is to apply for test shoots.

Test shoots

Test shoots are where photographers, models and make-up artists all get together and pool their resources. Models and photographers need 'Books' too, to enable *them* to get work. You should all end the session with some photographs for each of your Books. Some photographers may make a small charge to cover the studio fee, or may give you your photographs on disc and you will have to pay to have actual prints made for your Book. No one can afford to be out of pocket, so make sure you know exactly what you are getting in return for your services, before you go along to a test shoot. If you get one or two really good images for your Book, it will be a good day's work, even if there were no actual cash earnings involved.

Not all photographers are inexperienced photographers looking to put a Book together. Some professional photographers do test shoots routinely, to get work from agencies. A photographer may arrange a test shoot and inform a modelling agency, who may in turn send two or three inexperienced models (without Books) along for the session. The photographer would need a make-up artist on hand as it will be on the strength of his work, and the completed look of the model, that the agency may order photographs from him. Some take Polaroid photos of the shoot, and the models take these back to the agency. If the agency likes any of the Polaroid shots they will then buy a proper print to insert into the model's Book, which in turn may help her get work. Many of these young models have 'teenage' skin and you will find that the most important part of fashion make-up is to be able to do a perfect foundation – which appears flawless in the photograph. Remember, photographers *need* you!

Show reels

A fashion make-up artist will put together a Book of his or her best and most recent photographs to show prospective models. However, make-up artists working in film often have a show reel. A show reel is simply a moving portfolio of work either on video or a DVD. Just as fashion make-up artists will do test shoots to get photographs for their Book, film make-up artists may work on student films to get practice for film work. Instead of a print for their Book, they will receive a video of the film. The most important part of this film, apart from the make-up of course, is the mention the make-up artist will receive in the credits at the end of the film, stating his or her name as the make-up artist or the assistant.

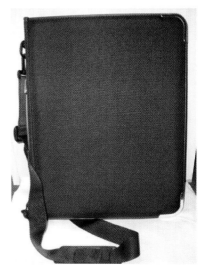

Suzanne's portfolio – closed

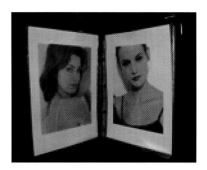

Suzanne's portfolio – open

AGENTS

Many make-up artists work freelance at the start of their careers to build up their Book and to gain experience. Many work as freelance artists because they also like the freedom it gives them, as they can organise family and other commitments around their work. Freelance make-up artists usually take on all kinds of make-up work, television, weddings, theatre and portraits. However, make-up artists working solely in fashion work usually need an agency to represent them.

KEY SKILLS

In all of the various branches of the make-up industry, there is one aspect that stands out and that is the necessity for 'people skills'. You must have a love of meeting and working with people, and you must be able to work as part of a team.

answers to knowledge review questions

Chapter One

1 Light colour is the light that comes from natural sources. Pigment colour is a substance that is capable of absorbing or reflecting light and of giving colour to the object it is applied to.

2 Mixing primary colours together would give you a dark brown to black colour.

3 Primary colours are pure colours, with no mixture of any other colour.

4 You can make tints and shades by either adding white or black respectively to a colour.

5 Brightness represents the range from light to dark.

6 Saturation is the level of purity of colour.

7 Harmony occurs when all chosen colours 'go well together'. Contrast is achieved by bringing together colours that are opposite each other in the chromatic circle 'colour wheel'.

8 To correct a red flushed face, green make-up concealer should be used.

9 To correct yellow undertones on a face, a purple concealer should be used.

10 The three colours traditionally known as primary colours are blue, red and yellow.

11 Secondary colours are colours mixed from two primary colours.

12 Warm colours are: red/orange. Cool colours are: blue/green.

13 Tertiary colours are colours mixed from a primary colour and a secondary colour.

14 Complementary colours are those which are opposite each other on the colour wheel.

15 An ashen skin tone is counteracted by a blue neutraliser.

16 Fill lights are a softer source of light often placed on the opposite side to a key light.

17 Top lighting, will create shadows underneath any bone structure, for example under the eyebrows, bags or lines under the eyes, nose to mouth lines, hollow cheeks and under the chin.

18 To achieve pictures that are sympathetic to the subject and comfortable to look at.

19 A light meter measures both the ambient light and the added effect of the flash head being used to illuminate the subject. Having measured the amount of light, the photographer will know how to adjust either the flash power or the camera to get the required exposure.

20 The photographer would use back lighting to create a feeling of space between the artist and the background.

Chapter Two

1 Activities you can do to achieve a professional appearance include: keep breath fresh; keep long hair tied back; keep nails short; wear comfortable shoes; keep own make-up minimal; keep deodorant wipes handy.

2 COSHH stands for Control of Substances Hazardous to Health.

3 The COSHH regulations provide guidance and lay down rules for the safe storage and use of potentially dangerous substances.

4 To make your working environment a safe place to work you can: make sure that all bottles and applicators are well labelled with full instructions if necessary; keep hazardous materials in a locked place; ensure that electrical sockets, plugs and all electrical equipment are checked regularly; replace anything with a frayed wire; dispose of any solvent removers safely in covered bins and always work in a well ventilated area.

5 To use a lipstick hygienically, always use a spatula to transfer the product onto a palette. From the palette use either a new disposable brush or an appropriate clean brush to apply the product.

6 To work efficiently, you should plan ahead – double check arrangements; check your make-up kit and make sure you do not run out of product; check your passport is not out of date, should you be working abroad; keep all continuity records.

7 You can organise your kit box by labelling everything clearly. Keep your fashion make-up separate from any theatrical/film make-up; organise in such a way that nothing gets damaged, spilt or broken. Anything potentially messy, should be wrapped in plastic bags, or cling film if necessary. Always keep any 'glitter' products totally separate from all other make-up.

8 Always keep some hand sanitisers in your kit box, in case there is no running water where you are working.

9 Items that should be stored separately in your make-up kit box are any potentially messy products like artificial blood or glycerine.

10 Cleaning solvents, isopropyl alcohol and surgical spirit, and other similar products cannot be stored in plastic bottles.

Chapter Three

1 The facial muscle corrugator draws the eyebrows together giving an expression of frowning.

2 The risorius muscles, found in the lower cheek, extending diagonally from the corners of the mouth, draw the corners of the mouth outwards giving an expression of smiling.

3 The three distinct layers of the skin are: the epidermis, the dermis and the subcutaneous layers.

4 Sebaceous glands produce sebum to lubricate the hair and the skin.

5 Contra indications to make-up/facial treatments include: bacterial/viral and fungal infections of eyes, lips or face; open cuts and abrasions; broken bones; acute acne and severe eczema or psoriasis.

6 Impetigo is a highly infectious skin disease that starts as small red spots, which then open up as blisters. It is most common around the corner of the mouth and if picked will spread. It can be spread through the use of dirty equipment.

7 Dry skin, sunburn, actinic keratosis and long-term changes in the skin's collagen.

8 Actinic keratosis appears as a persistent patch of scaly skin that has a pink, yellow, red or brownish tint.

9 Apply a sunscreen; use a sun block on your lips; choose a product that has been specially formulated for the lips, with a sun protection factor of 20 or more; limit your time outdoors when the sun is at its peak; wear sunglasses with UV light protection; wear light clothing that covers your arms and legs and a hat with a wide brim; be aware that some medications and skin-care products can increase your skin's risk of UV damage; and examine your entire skin surface thoroughly every month.

10 The general treatments for sunburn are cool compresses or misting the area with sprays of cool water. In extreme cases, a visit to the doctor may be required.

11 Cryosurgery is when the affected area is frozen with liquid nitrogen.

12 The best way to reduce the risk of non-melanoma skin cancer is to limit unprotected exposure to the sun, especially when the sun is at its most intense, generally 12–2 pm.

13 Basal-cell carcinomas usually develop on the skin of the face, chest, back and legs.

14 Squamous-cell carcinomas usually develop on sun-exposed skin, but can also occur on unexposed areas such as the external genitalia, fingers, toes and the soles of the feet.

15 Moles are spots on the skin – nearly everyone has them. They are made when skin cells called melanocytes grow in clusters, instead of being spread evenly throughout the skin.

16 Normal moles are evenly coloured and may or may not be raised. They have clear, even edges, and are usually circular or oval in shape.

17 The warning signs of the possible presence of melanoma in a mole are found in its asymmetry, border, colour and diameter.

18 Risk factors for sun-damaged skins, non-melanoma and melanoma skin cancers include: sun exposure; gender and age; fair skin and blue eyes; radiation exposure; reduced immunity; chemical exposure; genetic syndromes; and injury and inflammation.

19 A skin type described as combination is a combination of two or more skin types. The most common combination skin type is a greasy T-zone with a normal cheek area.

20 Black skin tends to wrinkle less because it contains more melanin, which is a powerful antioxidant, and because it has a thicker epidermis.

Chapter Four

1 Examples of sponges include the natural sponge, which is used for applying cake foundation with water to give a lightweight finish; soft sponges for liquid foundations; latex sponges, which are ideal for applying crème make-up; and hydra sponges, which are durable synthetic sponges suitable for most foundations.

2 A fan duster brush is a feather-fine duster used to gently remove excess setting powder. It can also help to soften the edges of make-up.

3 You would use an angled brush to give you precise angled application for eye shadow, eyeliner and eyebrows.

4 You would use a tapered point brush for glitter and for spot blending of creams and powders.

5 Tinted foundation, often called tinted moisturiser, offers a *very* light coverage. It is only used on very clear skin or to enhance a tan and is often used on young skin, but a very small amount can also be used as a male foundation.

6 The difference between standard make-up and camouflage make-up is that camouflage make-up has more pigment to give greater coverage of the skin. It is designed to disguise skin imperfections such as burns or scars but is extremely useful for covering unwanted freckles or liver spots caused by ageing. It is also used to cover tattoos.

7 Aqua colours are used for body and face painting.

8 Spirit gum is an adhesive used for applying false hair in theatrical make-up.

9 A stipple sponge is an open weave sponge used for creating a 'five o'clock shadow' beard, old age spots, bruises and other stippling effects.

10 Translucent powder is colourless.

11 To block out eyebrows you would use either an eyebrow wax or soap.

12 Disposable mascara brushes are recommended because it is difficult to sanitise the brush that comes with the mascara and avoid the dangers of cross-infection.

13 Titanium dioxide should be avoided on dark skins because they contrast too harshly with the natural skin colour, resulting in a grey appearance.

14 Lanolin is obtained from sheep's wool.

15 The two most common ingredients that may cause adverse reactions are preservatives and perfumes.

16 The purpose of sharpening lip and eyeliner pencils before each client is to give a clean uncontaminated surface to work with.

17 Lip glosses are made from mineral oils and pigments.

18 A frosted lipstick is a good recommendation for a model with very dry lips as it gives good durability as the product itself is very dry.

Chapter Five

1 There are five basic face shapes. They are oval, heart, round, long and square.

2 The 'perfect' face shape is commonly described as an oval face shape.

3 A heart shaped face is marked by being broad at the top and narrow at the bottom.

4 There are five basic eyebrow shapes: round, angled, soft angled, curved and flat.

5 Lip shapes include: thin, uneven, full, downward and mature.

6 It is necessary to complete a model consultation sheet to ascertain the client's requirements and expectations.

7 Clients may book into a beauty salon for a make-up application if they are looking for a complete change of look; for a special occasion make-up; for remedial camouflage make-up; or for a make-up lesson.

8 Immediate visual assessments include: checking foundation colour, checking eye and lip colour, the shape of the eyes and lips, the colour of the client's clothes, whether her hair style suits her, whether she has dark circles or bags under her eyes.

9 You should always assess the client's features sitting up, as facial features look very different when a model is lying flat.

10 Storyboards can show how a character develops throughout a TV or film production. They are useful if you are a make-up assistant standing in for the regular make-up artist. A soft copy storyboard can be easily distributed when the crew is international. Storyboards can also paint a thousand words.

11 A blank face make-up form is invaluable to list all the products used/to be used on the client.

12 It is important so that all the relevant details can be properly recorded in case someone else has to stand in for the regular make-up artist, for example an assistant.

Chapter Six

1 You would take an orange stick, or something similar, and draw a vertical line directly from the outside edge of the nostril upwards – this is where the inner edge of the eyebrow should start. Then join up the edge of the nostril to the outer edge of the eye – the continuing diagonal line will show you where the outer edge of the eyebrow should end.

2 The recommended time for eyebrow shaping and reshaping is 15 minutes and 30 minutes respectively.

3 The area should be cleansed and toned with antiseptic lotion, and the eyebrows brushed prior to the treatment.

4 You can minimise client discomfort during the eyebrow shaping treatment by grasping the hair by the surface of the skin and tweezing in the direction of hair growth.

5 The after care advice given to a client following an eyebrow shaping treatment is not to wear make-up for 12 hours after treatment.

6 The hygiene and safety precautions that should be followed when performing an eyebrow shape include: disposing of the removed hairs hygienically and sanitising the tweezers.

7 Contra indications that would prevent a permanent tinting treatment from being carried out include: a positive reaction to any product after a skin test; skin diseases or disorders including conjunctivitis, stye or blepharitis; viral infections – including a severe common cold; active eczema or psoriasis; contact lenses – unless removed; bruising to the eye area; and any inflammation or swelling around the eye.

8 If a model complains of irritation during an eyelash tinting treatment, remove the tint immediately with damp cotton wool pads, and irrigate the eye.

9 The developing time for eyelash tinting depends on the natural colour of the hair. Blond and fair hair develop rapidly, approximately 5 minutes. Red hair is more resistant and development can take longer, at approximately 10 minutes.

10 Eyelash perming should not be recommended when the lashes are fragile, the lashes are very short and sparse, or the lashes are naturally curly.

Chapter Seven

1 One sequence for applying make-up is: cleanse, tone, moisturise, then foundation, concealer, eyebrows, eyes, lips, powder, powder blusher and highlighting, contouring and shading.

2 If you have selected to do a smoky eye look, it may leave specks of colour over the cheeks. So foundation should be applied after eye shadow.

3 Specially formulated eye and lip primers can be used as an alternative to foundation.

4 You should use your largest brush to apply bronzer, as you do not want any hard lines.

5 You may need to create eyebrows if they have been blanked out with wax to create a particular look, if your model has no eyebrows due to illness or over tweezing.

6 The 'long eye' look is suited to close set eyes, as it widens their appearance with the eye shadow blending out towards the hairline.

7 Lip liners are used: to define the lips, to avoid the lipstick seeping out onto the skin and to help lip colour to last longer.

8 The best way to create the illusion of bigger lips is to use a medium tone lipstick or a creamy gloss.

9 An alternative to lip gloss is Vaseline.

10 The eyes will appear larger on a person wearing lenses for long sightedness.

Chapter Eight

1 The colour becomes irrelevant but the shade is apparent.

2 Photographic/beauty work needs to be perfect because the camera picks up every detail.

3 Learning the make-up fashions of past eras is important because all modern make-up has its roots in the past and you may be requested to re-create a particular look without time for research.

4 Black taffeta or leather patches were worn over skin imperfections in the seventeenth century.

5 Lips were small and rosebud shaped and painted red.

6 Queen Victoria had high moral standards and only stage actors and courtesans openly applied make-up. Women wore cosmetics, but with discretion. Painted faces were considered vulgar.

7 Women of the 1920s wanted to do something different following the strict moral code of the Victorian era before them, so they drank alcohol, smoked cigarettes and started to wear make-up abundantly.

8 The main features of a 1920s make-up are: a sad and wistful overall look with cupid's bow lips painted red and face pale and powdered.

9 The main features of a 1930s make-up were a porcelain base with translucent powder, white eye shadow and eyebrows concealed then re-designed in an arch shape using a pencil.

10 The two most apparent features of a 1950s make-up are the eyeliner flick and the red lipstick.

11 The main features of a 1960s make-up are the painted-in bottom lashes, smoky eyes and a pale foundation.

12 Bold colour and iridescent and frosted powders made the 1970s make-up different.

13 The early 1970s saw a 1920s revival in doll like features. The make-up company Biba hit on this for an advertising campaign.

14 Editorial work generally means close-up portrait work where very precise work is needed.

15 A 'story book' feature is one where the make-up on a model is adapted several times to produce different, but related looks.

16 The make-up for fashion shows/catwalks and pop videos can be described as developing very creative, cutting edge looks.

17 The Prada looks of 2002 and 2003 appeared as if no colour was used at all – just foundation and shine over the temples, although shading and highlighting were clearly used instead.

18 The long eye is particularly suitable for close set eyes, as the extended outer edge 'extends' the eye, making it look longer, which also makes it suitable for magazines.

19 The emphasis of the smoky eye look is that it is very dark and blended.

20 The make-up emphasis of catalogue work generally tends to be for natural, beautiful make-up.

Chapter Nine

1 The main aims of planning and promoting make-up activities are to promote the salon and to sell retail stock.

2 The main difference between a beauty salon make-up service and a cosmetics store make-up service is that in the beauty salon the model will apply make-up herself, whereas in a make-up store, the make-up artist will apply all the products.

3 The two ways to instruct a client who has come for a make-up lesson are either to give guidance and instruction and let the client do all the application herself, or to apply one half of the face and let the client complete the other half.

4 You should take a photograph of the model before the make-up lesson as the client often forgets how her make-up looked once the new look has been established.

5 You should allow sufficient time at the end of the make-up lesson to recommend retail items to the client.

6 The main health and safety consideration when unpacking stock is to dispose of all packaging safely.

7 The advantages of sending out invitations for group demonstrations are that the client feels special and is more likely to attend. Also, if you include an RSVP you will know how many people will be attending.

8 Holding a demonstration out of hours helps to make the clients you invite feel special and also allows you to concentrate on them and the demonstration without the distractions of day to day business.

9 You should ensure that you have sufficient stock at a group demonstration because it is almost inevitable that guests will want to buy products at the end of the event.

10 The items of information you need to know in advance of a fashion show include: how many models are involved, whether there will be a hairdresser, what type of clothes are being shown with how many changes, what is the age group of the models and audience, the location of the show, how many are expected in the audience, whether there will be space for a trade table at the show or an opportunity for you to hand out your own promotional material, and whether there will be posters advertising the event and/or TV coverage.

Chapter Ten

1 The six pieces of equipment used for making a paper pattern are: paper, pencil, ruler, record card with measurements, adhesive tape and scissors.

2 The record card is needed during pattern making for the measurements.

3 Circumference of head, ear to ear across the front hairline and nape.

4 The length of the paper pattern should be the circumference length.

5 The measurement used for the front hairline is temple to temple, or ear to ear.

6 The depth of the mount depends on the parting.

7 You ensure you have a perfect fit by placing the pattern onto the model's head to check the fit. Pleat where necessary and strengthen the edges with adhesive tape.

8 The main reason for a workroom order form is to keep a record of the client's details for items needed, including measurements of the head, client's personal details, type of postiche required and hair sample details. You include a hair sample with the workroom order form to ensure an exact match to client's own hair.

9 A photograph is helpful to the wigmaker to see exact hairline, any abnormalities that might be visible and the shape of the face.

10 Abnormalities include cysts and bumps.

Chapter Eleven

1 Wax is the product most often used in wound make-up. Waxes vary from soft wax through to eyebrow wax, which is a hard wax.

2 You would block out eyebrows to: conceal their colour; to flatten the hairs against the skin; and to remove, or to change the shape and/or size of the eyebrows. You may want to block out eyebrows for a specific look.

3 If eyebrow wax were not available, non-irritating soap could be used as a stand-by.

4 Sideburns, temple hair and front hairlines can also be blocked out with wax.

5 Red, blue, purple, yellow, brown and green are the colours of the bruise wheel.

6 Before creating a bullet wound, you would need to research what calibre gun was fired.

7 The two principal techniques of ageing are shading and highlighting.

8   Shading removes colour by taking back, causing the receding of shape.

9   Highlighting adds colour by bringing forward and making features stand out.

10 Bald caps are specifically made plastic caps intended to simulate a bald head.

11 Examples of custom made prosthetics are false ears, eye bags, swollen eye pieces, chins and noses.

12 Prosthetics are made from flexible materials like plastic, rubber or gelatine.

13 A life cast is a prosthetic piece that is made to measure for an individual model. First a mask is made to match the model and from this a duplicate positive casting is made with a material such as plaster or stone: this is called a face cast or body cast. From this a new shape is sculpted and is called a 'positive'.

14 When working with clay it should be kept wet and sealed inside a plastic bag.

15 The advantage of working with balsa wood is that it is versatile. It looks like bone, horn or steel and it can be carved, sanded, glued and painted.

16 Rigid Collodion is a safe product to use, whereas flexible Collodion contains harmful ingredients and should be avoided.

17 Grazes tend to occur on a bony prominence.

18 You would make a 'grit' effect by mixing coffee granules with a small amount of congealed blood paste.

19 Character make-up can be anything from simply adding a beard or moustache to applying the whole works – make-up, postiche and prosthetics.

20 With fictional or historical figures you need to research the age, health and temperament of the characters and aim to portray these in your make-up.

Chapter Twelve

1   Camouflage products differ from ordinary cosmetics in that they have: greater covering qualities; better holding power, designed to stay in place longer; resistance to the harmful rays of the sun; waterproofing; and a greater variety of colours for all ethnic skin tones.

2   Pigmentation and skin disorders that can be covered by camouflage make-up include port wine stains and other birthmarks, scars, tattoos, varicose veins, vitiligo and chloasma. Burns and disfigurements after surgery can also be covered using camouflage make-up.

3   The most important aspect of camouflage make-up is the ability to choose the correct colour to cover the imperfection. If the colour chosen is too light, it will look unnatural and pale, making the products look obvious, whereas if the colour is too dark, it will look fake.

4   A port wine stain is a flat, pink, red or purplish lesion usually caused by a blood vessel abnormality or capillary malformation of the skin. Port wine stains are usually on the face, but with correct camouflage make-up, they can be totally covered up.

5   'Faking faults' is necessary when the camouflaged area looks bland compared to the rest of the natural skin due to the absence of such conditions as freckles, moles, suntan, veins, capillaries, mottled redness, etc. on the skin, but not on the newly camouflaged areas. Simply copy the exact colour of the freckles, moles, etc. by random application over the camouflaged area using a brush or stipple sponge. Continue to create these 'faults' until a realistic effect is achieved.

6   Vitiligo is a pigmentation disorder in which melanocytes in the skin, the mucous membranes and the retina are destroyed. As a result, white patches of skin appear on different parts of the body, known as areas of de-pigmentation.

7   Vitiligo can be covered with stains, camouflage make-up or self-tanning lotions. Camouflaging is particularly effective for people whose vitiligo is on the face and hands.

8   Chloasma is a pigmentation disorder, usually appearing as brown patches, anywhere over the body, including the face. Its main cause is hormonal and it occurs most commonly in women, either during pregnancy or through the menopausal years or whilst taking the oral contraceptive pill.

9   Camouflage make-up can be used for people with chloasma. When choosing a foundation for someone with facial chloasma, do not be tempted to go too dark, to match the dark patch of de-pigmented skin – if anything this will just draw even more attention to the face. Choose

one shade darker than you would normally choose, and draw the attention to other areas of the face.

10 The main difference between a fashion make-up artist and a camouflage make-up artist is in the clients and models each different make-up artist will be making up. A fashion make-up artist will usually have young models, with a near perfect skin. A camouflage make-up artist's clients are likely to have a medical background. People with skin imperfections and pigmentation problems will make up the main part of their client base.

Chapter Thirteen

1 Do a product skin test on the model to ensure there were no adverse effects. Make sure the place of work is well ventilated, but warm. Have all equipment and products readily available and have the design sheet completed and agreed with the model.

2 Water colours, known as aqua paints are commonly used for face and body painting.

3 Brushes and sponges are used for face and body painting. These are usually larger than traditional make-up brushes, and the sponges are usually more porous.

4 The potential health hazard in airbrushing techniques is that the therapist and the model may breathe in a fine mist of paint.

5 Sponges used to create a stippling effect should be of an open texture. They are more porous allowing some of the paint to be stored inside the sponge.

6 There are two types of airbrush: dual action and single action.

7 It is appropriate to use airbrushing techniques when there are many models to make-up and for heavily scarred and imperfect skin it can add extra base to a specific area, no matter how small. It is also useful for prosthetic coverage. It will also be valuable for use on HDTV because the high number of pixels used will show any small imperfections.

8 You would make a stencil to create a repeat pattern.

9 The benefits of airbrushing are: it leaves the skin with a flawless finish, it can last 12–24 hours, it is lightweight, and it is undetectable even under close scrutiny.

10 You stop a vapour cloud formation when airbrushing by working in a well-ventilated environment or by using a filtered extractor fan.

Chapter Fourteen

1 Natural henna is obtained from leaves.

2 Three traditional uses for henna are weddings and bridal preparations, and the celebration of circumcision, pregnancy, birth and for general good luck, friendship and beauty.

3 Henna stains only the top layer of skin.

4 A skin test must be performed prior to a henna treatment to ensure that the model does not have any adverse reaction to the product being used.

5 Prior to a henna treatment, it is recommended that the model exfoliates the area to be designed.

6 On the treatment day, jewellery must be removed from the area, and a protective covering put over the model.

7 Contra indications to a henna treatment include cuts and abrasions and any skin disorders.

8 The usual breakdown of a henna recipe is 1 part henna powder, 2 parts liquid and $\frac{1}{2}$ part sugar.

9 You would know the henna powder had not been sifted if it contained small traces of sediment such as leaf stems and felt grainy between your fingers.

10 Mordents are chemical catalysts that help to activate the henna. Tamarind, coffee and tea are examples of mordents.

11 The minimum time which henna can take to develop is 2 hours.

12 After care advice includes: wearing loose clothing, keeping dry, avoid smudging immediately after the application and moisturising frequently after 12 hours.

13 There are four principal design styles in henna painting. These are Arabic, Indian, Sudanese and designs of self-expression.

14 Peacocks represent good luck.

15 Black henna should not be used as it contains a substance called paraphenylene diamine (PPD) which can cause severe dermatological problems.

glossary

Acetone a liquid solvent which melts plastic. It can be used for cleaning hair lace, but should never be used directly on the skin. Commonly, it is used for removing nail varnish. It is available from chemists.

Actinic keratosis pre-cancerous skin changes.

Albinism abnormal, non-pathological, partial or total absence of pigment in skin, hair and eyes.

Allergen a substance that causes an allergic reaction.

Antioxidants a substance that prevents a reaction with oxygen.

Astringents these contain a high percentage of alcohol. The ingredients used give varying effects such as the tightening sensation of antiperspirant products or a temporary reduction in pore size when used after cleansing on facial skin.

Basement membrane thin, extracellular layer consisting of basal lamina secreted by epithelial cells and reticular lamina secreted by connective tissue cells.

Biopsy removal of tissue or other material from the living body for examination, usually microscopic.

Blepharitis inflammation of the eye lid.

Brightness is the intensity of a colour, how dark or light it is.

Carcinoma a malignant tumour consisting of epithelial cells.

Chromatic brightness.

Coagulated refers to blood when blood clots have formed and has the appearance of being thick and jelly-like. Coagulation is the process by which a blood clot is formed.

Colour spectrum red, orange, yellow, green, blue, indigo, violet.

Comedones the correct term for blackheads.

Connective tissue the most abundant of the four tissue types in the body, performing the functions of binding and supporting; consists of relatively few cells in a great deal of intercellular substance.

Contra actions refers to negative reactions from a treatment or products, e.g. excessive erythema, allergic reactions.

Contra indications conditions or restrictions which indicate a particular service should not be carried out.

Cross infection transmitting infection from one person or surface to another.

Décolletage is a French word that describes the area from immediately below the chin, the neck and chest and the area covered when performing a facial massage.

Dermatosis papulosa nigra Lesions that develop through defects in the sebaceous follicles. They are benign, non-infectious but gradually increase in number.

Dermis the dermis is the deeper layer of the skin and its key functions are to provide support, strength and elasticity.

Desquamation the shedding of dead skin cells from the outer layer of the skin.

Discoid lupus erythematosus known as SLE (systemic lupus erythematosus); an auto-immune, inflammatory disease of connective tissue, occurring mostly in young women in their reproductive years.

Emollient a substance that soothes and softens the skin.

Emulsions these are products which contain both water and oil. Products can either be 'oil-in-water' products or 'water-in-oil' products, the difference being in the manufacturing stage.

Epidermal tissue refers to tissue from the epidermis.

Epidermis the epidermis is the most superficial layer of the skin and consists of five layers of cells. The three outermost layers consist of dead cells as a result of the process of keratinisation, the cells in the very outermost layer are dead and scaly and are constantly being rubbed away by friction.

Epidermodysplasia verruciformis an autosomal recessive trait with impaired cell-mediated immunity. About 15 human papilloma viruses are implicated in the associated infection, four of which lead to skin neoplasms. The disease begins in childhood with red papules and later spreads over the body as grey and yellow scales.

Erythema redness to the skin caused by irritation, or injury to the tissue.

Ferrule the metal end of a make-up brush that forms the joint between the hairs and the wooden handle and helps to strengthen the brush.

Foundation (in wig and postiche making) is the base of any piece of postiche. Made of net, to which hair is attached.

Free radicals these lead to out-of-control oxidation which damages healthy cells.

Glycerine oily liquid, which can be used for sweat, or lymph on a burn, for example. Can be bought from most high-street chemists. The technical term for glycerine is glycerol.

Greasepaint another word for cream make-up.

Hackle/Hackling a tool used in combing and mixing loose hair. Constructed of metal spikes set in a wooden block, it is rather like a miniature bed of nails. The action of mixing the hair is known as hackling.

Hair lace a very fine flesh-coloured mesh used to blend off hairlines where they meet the skin to give a natural hairline effect. The fine lace is covered with make-up. Mainly used for screen and the theatre.

Hue the term used for stand-alone colours: red, blue, green, etc.

Hygiene requirements the standard expected, as laid down in law, industry codes of practice, or written procedures specified by the organisation.

Hypothyroidism a condition describing an under-active thyroid gland.

Inorganic pigments pigments usually obtained from chemical sources.

Irritant any substance, usually chemical, that can cause simple to severe irritation to the skin or mucus membranes.

Keloids the formation of excess collagen in the form of thick interlacing bundles which causes marked swelling at the site of the wound.

Keratinised/keratinisation the process by which the cells become horny due to their deposition of keratin within them.

Lanolin a yellowish viscous wax obtained by refining the wool grease that is secreted by the sebaceous glands of sheep.

Legislation laws affecting the conduct of business, treatments, the premises or working environment, people employed and systems of work.

Life casting/cast technique of taking an impression of a section or piece of an actor's face or body and casting it in stone.

Mastication a term that refers to chewing.

Mastoid process a 'process' is any prominent projection. The mastoid process is a rounded projection of the temporal bone posterior to the external auditory meatus. It serves as a point of attachment for several neck muscles.

Melanin produced by cells called melanocytes. Melanin is a dark black, brown or yellow pigment found in some parts of the body such as the skin.

Mitosis the orderly division of the nucleus of a cell that ensures that each new daughter nucleus has the same number and kind of chromosomes as the original parent nucleus. The process includes the replication of chromosomes and the distribution of the two sets of chromosomes into two separate and equal nuclei.

Networking building contacts with many other people in the industry.

Neutraliser to neutralise something is to make it chemically or electrically neutral. In this instance, however, a neutraliser is a product that removes colour from the skin, taking it back to a more natural colour. Green for example, will lessen redness and therefore is known as a neutraliser.

Nevoid Basal Cell Carcinoma Syndrome a form of cancer characterized by the appearance of lesions and the development of multiple cysts and bony formations of the face and head. The lesions may be found on the first layer of the skin (epidermis) or in the mucous membranes of the mouth. The connective tissues and the nervous and vascular (blood vessel) systems of the body may also be affected. The skin lesions are limited in size, and are not usually due to any external causes.

Nuclei the plural for nucleus and the largest structure within a cell. It contains the hereditary factors of the cell, called genes, which control cellular structure and direct many cellular activities. Most body cells contain a single nucleus, although some, such as mature red blood cells, do not. Skeletal muscle fibres (cells) contain several nuclei.

Organisational requirements beauty therapy procedures or work rules issued by the salon management.

Panchromatic sensitive to all colours.

Papillary layer found in the dermis its key function is to provide vital nourishment to the living layers of the epidermis above.

Personal appearance hair is secured away from the face or an appropriate length and style so as not to interfere with the treatment. Nails are clean, free of varnish and of a suitable length so as not to interfere with the treatment. The only permitted jewellery is a wedding band and small unobtrusive earrings. Shoes should be clean, low heeled and fit securely around the foot. Uniforms should be freshly laundered.

Photo-ageing premature ageing of the skin because of sun exposure.

Postiche a French word used to describe all added hairpieces. The pieces can be as small as a false eyelash or as large as a wig. Postiche work for the face comprises of beards, moustaches, sideburns and eyebrows.

Preservatives substances added to products to give them a longer shelf life. Most preservatives are chemically based, but there are natural preservatives like the vitamins A, C and E, which are all antioxidants.

Prosthetics custom made prosthetics are 3D pieces designed to alter the shape of a face or body for use in theatre and television for horror or fantasy effects. Examples include false ears, eye bags, swollen eye pieces, chins and noses. Usually they are made of latex or plastic and can be fixed in position with spirit gum, or other suitable adhesives.

Relevant person an individual deemed responsible for supervising you during a given task or service, or the person to whom you normally report.

Reticular layer found in the dermis and lies beneath the papillary layer, having the same functions.

Rubber mask A castor-oil based product, available in various colours, used for painting on top of latex.

Sanitisation refers to cleansing or washing to an antiseptic level so as to inhibit bacteria.

Saturation the level of purity of a colour.

Senile purpura increased fragility of the skin's blood vessels due to a combination of ageing and sun exposure.

Shade made by mixing black with a colour.

Silicone one of the many polymeric organic compounds of silicon with high resistance to cold, heat, water and the passage of electricity.

Skin sensitivity tests determine the degree of skin reaction and sensitivity.

Sterilisation the total destruction of all micro-organisms.

Stippling technique of using an open-pored sponge and applying make-up with a dabbing movement in order to provide a textured effect.

Structural collagen a protein that is the main organic constituent of connective tissue.

Subcutaneous a thick layer of connective tissue found below the dermis. The subcutaneous layer of skin contains the same collagen and elastin fibres as the dermis and also contains the major arteries and veins that supply the skin, forming a network throughout the dermis.

Systemic medical condition a medical condition caused by a defect in one of the body organs, e.g. the heart and lungs.

Teasing the manual loosening of entangled hair before hackling.

Threading this is a method of hair removal which is practised in Asia and Europe. A piece of cotton thread is rolled over the area of unwanted hair, which causes the hairs to twist around it. The technician then pulls on the thread, which, in turn, pulls the hairs caught around it out by the root. Threading should be done only by a highly skilled professional.

Tint made by mixing white with a colour

Titanium dioxide an inorganic oxide that comes in the form of a white powder. It is used chiefly in colour cosmetics, but it is also used in sunscreens.

Tone created by mixing colours; it can range from almost pure colour (hue) to grey.

Toxin refers to substances that are poisonous to the human body.

Treatment plan the stage or plan you intend to follow in carrying out a particular treatment. The basic contents of a treatment plan include: areas to be treated, type of treatment, known contra indications, contra actions, treatment advice, client signature, client feedback.

Tumour a growth of excess tissue due to an unusually rapid division of cells.

Tuplast thick substance in a tube that is squeezed onto the skin to simulate blisters. Can also be used for modelling scars on the skin. Press the skin together around the Tuplast, and blow-dry with cold air from a hairdryer.

Urea a substance found in urine – the fluid produced by the kidneys that contains wastes or excess materials and is excreted from the body through the urethra. Small amounts of urea can also be found in sweat.

Xeroderma pigmentosum a rare inherited (autosomal recessive) disease in humans associated with increased sensitivity to ultraviolet induced mutagenesis and thus skin cancer. Sensitivity can be demonstrated in cultured cells and appears to be due to deficiency in DNA repair, specifically in excision of ultraviolet induced thymine dimers. Afflicted individuals are extremely sensitive to light and develop eye and skin abnormalities such as premature ageing, keratoses and skin cancers and must be kept completely away from UV light.

Zygomatic process a 'process' is any prominent projection. The zygomatic process consist of two zygomatic bones commonly referred to as the cheekbones, and form the prominences of the cheeks.

resources

Le Quesne Academy – Fashion & Photographic Make-Up Schools (UK)
Academia Le Quesne – Fashion & Photographic Make-Up Schools (Spain)
e-mail: enquiries@lequesne-enterprises.com
www.lequesne-enterprises.com

The Le Quesne Academy is a highly respected training centre for fashion and photographic make-up, beauty and holistic therapies, and is an approved assessment centre for Vocational Training Charitable Trust (VTCT). Fashion make-up is a precise art – form and accuracy and precision are the key words for their courses. Several courses are offered: one-day refresher courses, five-day intensive courses and a four-

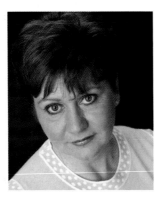

Suzanne Le Quesne

week intensive Fashion and Photographic Make-Up Diploma course – which is second to none. Unique to the diploma course is the photographic evidence students start collecting from day one, taken with digital cameras on-site in training locations. On the four-week intensive course, students get the opportunity to take part in photo shoots and meet and work with professional photographers and models. They leave with four good quality prints (black and white and colour) in a personalised leather portfolio provided with the course, to start them on their professional career.

The Le Quesne Academy also provides student make-up starter kits for Level 2 make-up. Everything students need in a starter-kit to fulfil NVQ Level 2 Make-Up modules. An extensive range of excellent quality make-up from The Le Quesne Collection, each item individually selected by Suzanne Le Quesne. See website for full details. Generous discounts for college orders.

Suzanne is happy to visit colleges, to give talks or demonstrations, to show students her professional portfolio, or to judge make-up competitions. Please e-mail any enquiry.

Anthony Braden Cosmetics Ltd
P O Box 576
Woking, Surrey
GU23 7YE, United Kingdom
Tel: (44) 01483 213005
Fax: (44) 01483 211685
e-mail: sales@anthonybraden.co.uk
www.anthonybraden.co.uk

Anthony Braden Cosmetics provide a wide range of make-up products, a world class natural manicure system and quality brushes for students, therapists and professional beauty salons. These products are designed to be used in a professional capacity within a salon or spa and then to be sold on to the general public.

They provide CPD (Continued Professional Development) Training under the guidance of our Director of Education, Suzanne Le Quesne.

In addition they supply student make-up starter kits and manicure kits, for all students of Level 2 make-up. They are happy to visit a college or salon to discuss your requirements. Please phone in the first instance.

The Bakery – Digital Photographic Studios
Advance Park
Wrexham
LL14 3YR
Tel: 01978 823000
e-mail: myk@BigLoaf.com
www.BigLoaf.com

The Bakery digital photographic studio is a foundation to promote the awareness, interest and training in the visual arts and related crafts. The Bakery offers five studios, exhibition space and photography training. They will do everything to support client's requirements providing any or all of the equipment needed.

If you are an aspiring model, or a make-up student looking to build a fashion or theatrical portfolio, they can help you. The Bakery prides itself in having the very best facilities to be found in any photographic studio.

Three Kings Make-Up
Showroom and Studio
84 Queens Road
North Camp
Farnborough
Hampshire, GU14 6JR
Phone: (+44) 01252 371123
Fax: (+44) 01252 515516
e-mail: info@threekingstheatrical.com
www.thethreekingstheatrical.com

'Three Kings Make-up'
is part of The Three
Kings Theatrical
Supply Group. This is
a family run business
offering a wide range
of theatrical services,
but specialising in
professional make-up.

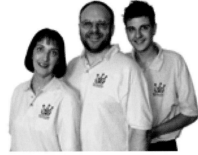

The Three Kings

They hold a large
range of make-up
from most of the
leading brands, including Ben Nye, Grimas, Leichner, Face to
Face (Make-Up International), Mehron, Snazaroo, Stargazer,
Temptu and others, as well as their own range of casualty
simulation make-up products. All of their make-up is 10%
below the recommended retail price, with no minimum
order.

Clients come from a wide sector, including TV, stage, film,
amateur dramatic groups, first aid training organisations, face
painters, clowns, transgender and many more.

A large modern training studio is available for hire. VTCT
(Vocational Training Charitable Trust) accredited courses and
other training sessions, including casualty simulation and
airbrushing, are run on a regular basis.

See website for details of make-up equipment and
accessories, including a wide range of make-up boxes.

The MOLE Clinic
222 Regent Street
London W1B 5TR
Phone: 020 7297 2075
www.themoleclinic.co.uk

The MOLE Clinic is the UK's leading skin cancer screening
clinic.

Featuring the award winning microDERM® Expert System for
Advanced Screening for Skin Cancer, their systems capture
highly magnified digital images of moles, allowing their team
of highly trained nurses to *look inside* a mole and spot signs
of even early melanoma. Mole images are then analysed by
analytical software, and allocated a Melanoma Risk Score –
a highly accurate predictor of melanoma skin cancer.

The MOLE Clinic also offers the removal of suspect moles,
and normal moles for purely cosmetic reasons, by top
surgeons.

Clinics throughout the UK.

SkinCeuticals
10 Gordon Road,
London W5 2AD
Phone: 020 8997 8541
e-mail: sales@skinceuticals.co.uk
www.skinceuticals.co.uk

Did you know that using a Vitamin-C formulation can be one
of the most effective ways to prevent premature ageing and
environmental damage to your skin? The SkinCeuticals
research team helped pioneer the advent of 'cosmeceuticals'
with the development of a topical vitamin C formula that is
scientifically proven to protect skin from premature signs of
ageing caused by environmental damage.

The brand uses pure, pharmaceutical grade ingredients with
proven scientific results. Formulations are based on optimal
concentrations of active ingredients that are elegantly crafted
into functional products designed, formulated and tested for
effectiveness.

The brand's dedication to developing advanced skin care
backed by science has earned SkinCeuticals a strong
reputation with the world-wide medical community.
Thousands of dermatologists, skin care professionals,
cosmetic surgeons and medi-spas in 35 countries trust Skin
Ceuticals to promote skin health. There are now more than
100 stockists across the UK and Ireland.

Aroosa Beauty Salon and Training Centre
Shabana Begum
Phone: 07866 351117
e-mail: aroosabeauty@hotmail.com

All aspects of hair and beauty covered: weddings and
photographic make-overs, bridal hair and henna specialist.
Airbrush trainer for Impet2us Limited.

Judie Becque
Make-Up Artist
e-mail: judie.becque@btinternet.com

Ann Eatwell
Face and Body Painter
Phone: 07867 910984
e-mail: ann@catchacolour.com
www.catch-a-colour.com

Specialising in body painting, theatrical make-up and
children's face painting.

Ema Doherty – Make-Up Artist/College Lecturer
E M A – Exact Make-up Art
For make-up, hair and airbrush services
Phone: 07976 661702
e-mail: ema@exactmakeupart.co.uk
www.exactmakeupart.co.uk

Impet2us Limited
UK distribution and training academy for Temptu
Phone: 01386 765363
e-mail: info@impet2us.co.uk
www.impet2us.co.uk

Suppliers of airbrush make-up, airbrush equipment, temporary tattoos, body paints, eyebrow stencils and airbrush training.

Donna Jones
Camouflage Make-Up Artist
e-mail: beautybydonna@wales34.freeserve.co.uk
www.geocities.com/beautybydonna

Sue Kennedy
Make-Up Artist
Tel: 07759 329190
e-mail: slcallaghan@hotmail.com

Adéle Palmer
Fashion Make-Up Artist
e-mail: adele_palmer@yahoo.co.uk

Tamsin Pyne
Fashion Make-up Artist
e-mail: mamstin@hotmail.com

Paula Southern
Face Painting Artist
paula@amazingfaces.co.uk
www.amazingfaces.co.uk

Dorinda Sweales
Make-Up Artist/College Lecturer
e-mail:dorinda@dizzyheightsmakeup.co.uk
www.dizzyheightsmakeup.co.uk

Vanessa Wayne
Creative Photographer
Tel: 01252 660701
Fax: 01252 404590
e-mail: vanessa@photoness.co.uk
www.creativeglamour.co.uk
www.photoness.co.uk

As well as working as a creative photographer, Vanessa also creates beautiful wedding photography.

bibliography

Baker, Patsy, *Wig making and Make-up for Theatre Television and Film*, Focal Press, 1993.

Brown, Bobbi, with Sally Wadyka, *Bobbi Brown Beauty Evolution*, Aurum, 2003.

Charlwood, Maurene, and Cheryl Robertson, *Cosmetic Watch*, Elliot Right Way Books, 2001.

Corson, Richard, *Fashions in Makeup – From Ancient to Modern Times*, Peter Owen, 2003.

Musgrove, Jan, *Media Make-up. Hair and Costume for Film and Television*, Focal Press, 2003.

Nordmann, Lorraine, *Beauty Therapy – The Official Guide to Level 2*, Cengage Learning, 1995.

index